Fueling The

Teen Machine

SECOND EDITION

Ellen L. Shanley, MBA, RD, CD-N

Colleen A. Thompson, MS, RD

University of Connecticut

Bull Publishing Company
Boulder, Colorado

Copyright © 2011 by Bull Publishing Company

Bull Publishing Company
P.O. Box 1377
Boulder, CO 80306
www.bullpub.com
800-676-2855

ISBN 978-1-933503-37-0

Distributed to the trade by:
Independent Publishers Group
814 North Franklin Street
Chicago, IL 60610

Manufactured in the United States of America

Library of Congress Cataloging-in-Publication Data

Shanley, Ellen L.
Fueling the teen machine/Ellen L. Shanley, Colleen A. Thompson—2nd ed.
    p. cm.
Includes bibliographical references and index.
ISBN 978-1-933503-37-0
1. Teenagers—Nutrition. 2. Physical fitness for children. 3. Physical fitness—Nutritional aspects. 4. Cooking. I. Thompson, Colleen A. II. Title.

RJ235.S52 2011
613.7'043—dc22   2010035112

Publisher: James Bull
Production: Publication Services
Composition: Shadow Canyon Graphics
Cover design: Lightbourne Images

10 9 8 7 6 5 4 3 2 1

Contents

iii

Acknowledgments

We would like to take this opportunity to thank our families and colleagues for their continued support. Taking on a project like this is not easy.

Ellen would like to thank her husband, Peter, for always being agreeable and supportive, and her two children, Amanda and Gregg, for putting up with some craziness.

Colleen would like to thank her husband, Brian, for his unending support and her three wonderful boys, Alex, Kevin, and Eric, for helping her to always find the balance in her life.

We feel fortunate to be at the University of Connecticut in the Department of Allied Health Sciences in the College of Agriculture and Natural Resources. The support of our department head, Lawrence Silbart, Ph.D., as well as of the entire dietetics faculty makes it easier to be successful and productive.

Thank you all—we couldn't have done it without you.

— Ellen and Colleen

Preface

Okay, so you're not really a machine.

Your body does work like a machine, though. You've got to keep all the parts in working order, inside and out, and put the right fuel in so that it is efficient and lasts for years. No cars last forever, but some get better mileage and last longer than others. This book is designed to help you make the most of the model you have. You can't trade in your model, but you can improve it, tune it, and keep it in shape to last a long time and feel terrific.

The fact that you've even picked up this book says that you're interested in knowing what it takes to lead a healthy, active life, choosing nutritious (and tasty.) foods. Hopefully, you'll do more than just pick up this book—you'll read it, enjoy it, and refer to it many times.

We've updated the book to include the latest information on a host of topics ranging from sports nutrition to eating disorders to vegetarianism. Things have certainly changed since our first edition was published. This edition includes a chapter on physical activity, and more information on organic foods, "superfoods," and the latest scoop on fast food facts. You can find out the best websites to visit and even learn how to plan a menu! We've included the most current information on the Dietary Guidelines, the Food Guide Pyramid and the Dietary Reference Intakes. For you techies, we encourage you to download some cool apps for your phone that can track your fitness progress or tell you the calorie content in your favorite restaurant meal. Finally, there are some tasty recipes that we know you will enjoy! The recipes are easy and healthy with lots of "superfoods"! So take your time and enjoy the book. We hope you will enjoy reading it and will apply your newly learned facts to a healthy active lifestyle as a teenager!

Each chapter stands alone, but you'll probably want to read all of them to really arm yourself with the facts for "fueling your body."
So start up your engines, and let's go.

The Basics

The teenage years are a busy time. You've got school, homework, after-school activities, things to do with friends and family, chores around the house, maybe even a job. Whew. With all there is to do, it's hard to find time to pay attention to what you eat. Yet, the one way to juggle all those responsibilities is to have enough energy to do them all (or at least as many as you want to.). How do you get that energy? Eat.

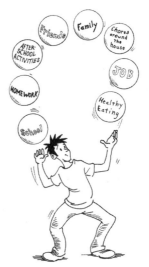

You're probably thinking, "Eat? That's easy. I already do that." You're right. It can be easy—if you have the right information to help you make choices. Eating is really all about choices. Nowadays there are so many choices that it can be hard to know where to start. The supermarkets seem to showcase new products every day. The labels use terms such as "lite," "lean," "low-fat," "nonfat," "organic," and "low-carb." The stores are full of new books on nutrition, the latest diets, supplements, sports nutrition, and a host of other topics. There's the Internet and infomercials for health and nutrition products. How can you sort through all the information out there and make any sense of it for yourself and for what *you* need? We're going to help you do that. The best place to start is with some basic nutrition guidance. The best source for that is the Dietary Guidelines for Americans.

Every five years or so, the U.S. Department of Agriculture and the Department of Health and Human Services issue the Dietary Guidelines for Americans. The latest guidelines were issued in 2005. Their mission is "to provide positive, simple and consistent messages to help consumers achieve healthy, active lifestyles." The guidelines are general in nature, allowing consumers (that includes you) choice and flexibility when it comes to their diet. As of this book going to press, the 2010 guidelines were not released. We do know that the emphasis will be similar to that in the 2005 guidelines, including whole grains, increased fruit and vegetable consumption, and balancing food intake with physical activity.

The *Dietary Guidelines for Americans 2005* provide "science-based advice to promote health and to reduce risk for major chronic diseases through diet and physical activity." Unfortunately, the major causes of sickness and even death in the United States today are related to a poor diet and being physically inactive. These diseases include heart disease, diabetes, and certain cancers. In addition, poor diet and physical inactivity cause an energy imbalance. This means that we are eating more calories than we are using. This can cause overweight and obesity. So the newest Dietary Guidelines emphasize eating the right amount of calories and getting plenty of physical activity. For detailed information on the Dietary Guidelines you can visit the website at www.health.gov/dietaryguidelines/. Below is a summary of the guidelines and key recommendations.

ADEQUATE NUTRIENTS WITHIN CALORIE NEEDS

Key Recommendations

- Eat a variety of foods and beverages from all of the food groups.
- Choose foods that are lower in fat, saturated fat, trans fats, cholesterol, added sugars, and salt. Use "MyPyramid" to help you

choose a balanced diet that has enough calories and nutrients from all of the food groups.

WEIGHT MANAGEMENT

Key Recommendations

- To maintain body weight in a healthy range, balance the calories that you eat from food and beverages with the calories that you use being active.
- To prevent gradual weight gain over time, make small decreases in food and beverage calories and increase your physical activity.

PHYSICAL ACTIVITY

Key Recommendations

- Get plenty of physical activity and reduce sedentary activities to promote health, psychological well-being, and a healthy body weight.
- Your physical activity should include some cardiovascular activity, such as running, playing basketball or soccer, or any activity that gets your heart rate going. Add some stretching for flexibility and resistance or strength exercises for muscle and bone strength and endurance.
- Teens should aim for at least 60 minutes of physical activity on most, preferably all, days of the week.

FOOD GROUPS TO ENCOURAGE

Key Recommendations

- Eat enough fruits and vegetables while staying within energy needs. Two cups of fruit and 2½ cups of vegetables per day are a good start for someone eating about 2,000 calories each day.

- Try to vary the fruits and vegetables that you eat each day. Choose from all five vegetable subgroups (dark green, orange, legumes, starchy vegetables, and other vegetables) several times a week.
- Eat at least three or more 1-ounce equivalents of whole-grain products per day, with the rest of the recommended grains coming from enriched or whole-grain products. In general, at least half of the grains should come from whole grains (more information on whole grains in Chapter 2).
- Eat or drink at least 3 cups per day of fat-free or low-fat milk or equivalent milk products, such as cheese or yogurt.

FATS

Key Recommendations

- Eat less than 10 percent of calories from saturated fatty acids and less than 300 mg/day of cholesterol, and keep trans fatty acids in your diet as low as possible.
- Keep total fat intake between 20 to 35 percent of calories, with most fats coming from sources of healthy fatty acids, such as fish, nuts, and vegetable oils.
- For children and teens aged 4–18, the recommendation is 25–35% of calories from fat.
- When selecting and preparing meat, poultry, dry beans, and milk or milk products, make choices that are lean, low-fat, or fat-free.
- Limit intake of fats and oils high in saturated and/or trans fatty acids, and choose products low in such fats and oils.

CARBOHYDRATES

Key Recommendations

- Choose fiber-rich fruits, vegetables, and whole grains often.
- Choose and prepare foods and beverages with little added sugars or caloric sweeteners.

- Reduce your incidence of cavities by practicing good oral hygiene and eating sugar- and starch-containing foods and beverages less frequently.

SODIUM AND POTASSIUM

Key Recommendations

- Consume less than 2,300 mg (approximately 1 teaspoon of salt) of sodium per day.
- Choose and prepare foods with little salt. At the same time, consume potassium-rich foods, such as fruits and vegetables.

FOOD SAFETY

Key Recommendations

- To avoid microbial foodborne illness, do the following:

  - Clean hands, food contact surfaces, and fruits and vegetables. Meat and poultry should not be washed or rinsed.
  - Separate raw, cooked, and ready-to-eat foods while shopping, preparing, or storing foods.
  - Cook foods to a safe temperature to kill microorganisms.
  - Chill (refrigerate) perishable food promptly and defrost foods properly.
  - Avoid raw (unpasteurized) milk or any products made from unpasteurized milk, raw or partially cooked eggs or foods containing raw eggs, raw or undercooked meat and poultry, unpasteurized juices, and raw sprouts.

MyPyramid

The Dietary Guidelines are pretty general in nature, as you can see. To get more specific information on *what and how much* to eat, you can check out MyPyramid. The pyramid is a way to put the Dietary Guidelines into practice. What is neat about the pyramid is that it is designed to be personalized. In other words, one size does not fit all. You may need a different amount of calories and different number of servings of fruits and vegetables than your best friend. After all, no two people are exactly alike, right?

MyPyramid offers personalized eating plans and interactive tools to help you plan and assess your food choices based on the Dietary Guidelines for Americans. You'll need to use the Internet to personalize your pyramid: go to www.mypyramid.gov. Once you're there, you can click on "Personalize MyPyramid" plan. Enter your gender, height, weight, and activity level. Then your personalized plan is created. You can even listen to podcasts, plan a healthy menu, and look up foods and play games.

So let's look more closely at this pyramid. You can see from Figure 1.1 (see the color insert immediately following page 40) that the pyramid has several colored striped sections. Each section is a different size, and each section represents a different food group. Let's take a quick look at each food group and talk about what is most important to know about each of these groups.

Grains

The biggest section of the pyramid is the orange section for grains. The advice for grains is pretty simple: Eat at least 3 ounces of whole-grain bread, cereals, rice or pasta every day.

Look for the word "whole" before the grain name on the list of ingredients on the food label (see Chapter 12 to learn more about the food label). Why are whole grains better? Whole grains have more fiber, vitamins, and minerals than simple or processed grains. The fiber in whole grains helps make you feel full and eat less. When choosing bread, look for "whole grain" on the label. We talk more about grains in Chapter 2, Finding Your Fuel.

Table 1.1 How to Use MyPyramid		
FOOD GROUP/ SERVING SIZE	**WHY SHOULD I?**	**HOW COULD I?**
Grains Approximately 5-7 ounces per day for most teens; make half of your servings whole grain An ounce is 1 slice of bread, 1 ounce of cereal, ½ cup pasta	Good sources of fiber, B vitamins, of fiber, B vitamins, iron, magnesium, zinc.	1 ounce whole-grain cereal for breakfast 2 ounces whole-grain bread for sandwich with lunch Snack: 6 crackers ½ cup pasta or rice with dinner Total = 5 servings (3 whole-grain)
Vegetables 2-3 cups/day for most teens Choose dark green, leafy veggies and deep orange veggies raw chopped vegetables	Vegetables provide essential vitamins essential vitamins such as vitamin A, vitamin C, and folate. They also provide fiber and some minerals.	½ cup raw carrot sticks with lunch ½ cup leafy green lettuce and tomato on your sandwich 1 cup cooked veggies with dinner Total = 2 cups
Fruits (1½-2 cups/day for most teens Choose whole fresh fruit as much as possible Vary your fruits	Fruits give us vitamins A and C and are good sources of fiber	¾ cup fruit juice at breakfast 1 cup berries with lunch Snack on 1 medium apple Total = 3 cups

(continued on next page)

Table 1.1 How to Use MyPyramid (cont)		
FOOD GROUP/ SERVING SIZE	**WHY SHOULD I?**	**HOW COULD I?**
Milk 3 cups/day Choose low-fat or skim milk, yogurt, cheese	This group provides calcium, vitamin D, protein, and riboflavin.	½ cup low-fat milk on cereal = ½ milk serving 1 cup yogurt with lunch 1 ounce string cheese snack = ½ milk serving 1 cup low-fat milk with dinner Total = 3 cups
Meat and beans 5-6 ounces/day for most teens All foods made from meat, poultry, fish, dry beans, or peas, eggs, nuts, and seeds are considered part of this group. Dry beans (such as kidney beans, black beans, or garbanzo beans) and peas are part of this group as well as part of the vegetable group.	This group provides lots of protein as well as iron, niacin, vitamin B-6, vitamin B-12, and zinc.	2 ounces lean turkey for lunch 3 ounces lean meat for dinner ¼ cup almonds for snack Total = 5½ ounces

Table 1.1 How to Use MyPyramid (cont)		
FOOD GROUP/ SERVING SIZE	**WHY SHOULD I?**	**HOW COULD I?**
Oils 5 teaspoons/day for most teens Choose healthier oils, such as olive oil, canola oil, and the oil in nuts and fish. Solid fats from butter, margarine, and fatty meats are less healthy choices, so go easy on these.	Provide essential fatty acids necessary for health	2 teaspoons mayonnaise on sandwich 3 teaspoons salad dressing (made with olive or canola oil) with dinner Total = 5 teaspoons

Vegetables

The next section of the pyramid is the green section for vegetables. The advice for vegetables is "vary your vegetables." You should try to eat plenty of vegetables every day and choose different vegetables as much as possible. The more color there is in your vegetables, especially dark green and orange, the better they are for you.

- Eat more dark green veggies (such as spinach, broccoli, and kale)
- Eat more orange veggies (such as carrots and sweet potatoes)
- Eat more beans and peas; they have lots of fiber.

Fruits

The red section of the pyramid is for the fruit group. Focus on fruit. Eat lots of fruit every day, and, just as with the vegetables, try to eat different varieties of fruit. Go easy on the fruit juice and focus on whole fruits. You'll get more fiber that way and less sugar. Oranges, apples, and bananas are great, but why not try to include more blueberries, strawberries, and cantaloupe, too. Nowadays, there are many exotic fruits available year-round right in your local supermarket. Try a mango or a kiwi for something new.

Milk and Milk Products

The blue section of the pyramid is for the milk group. Teens are still growing, and their bones are still growing, too. The calcium and vitamin D in milk and milk products really help you build and keep your bones strong and healthy. You need to drink plenty of milk every day, at least 3 cups. Low-fat and skim milk are just fine and taste great. You can choose low-fat yogurt, cheeses, and ice cream as well.

Meat and Beans

The purple strip on the pyramid is for meat and beans. Choose lean cuts of meat, poultry, and fish. Bake, broil, and grill your meat to keep it lean and tasty. Nuts and beans fall into this group, too. Almonds, peanuts, and cashews make a great snack that is packed with protein. Just watch the portion size, because it is easy to eat more than you need.

Fats and Oils

The thin yellow strip on the pyramid represents the group from which you need the least amount each day—fats and oils. Everyone needs a little bit of fat for the essential fatty acids. But some fats are better for you than others (see Chapter 2, Finding Your Fuel). Choose healthier fats, such as olive oil, canola oil, and the oil in nuts and fish. Solid fats from butter, margarine, and fatty meats are less healthy and should be limited in your diet.

Discretionary Calories

Finally, the pyramid refers to something called "discretionary calories." These are food choices that are "extras" in the diet, including sweets, desserts, fried foods, sweetened drinks such as soda, etc. These foods can be part of your diet, but they need to be consumed in limited amounts. That's because they don't really give you much in the way of vitamins, minerals, or fiber. They mostly just give you extra calories—that you may not need. It's all about choices. Make your choices count.

Be sure to visit the MyPyramid website to find out more about your personalized pyramid plan (for some quick info, check out Table 1.1). There are also lots of interactive tools, games, and menu planners there. You can have fun and learn a little something at the same time.

Mind you, no one can be perfect when it comes to eating. Who needs to be? All foods can certainly fit into a healthy diet. It's really about choices and portions of foods. You needn't deprive yourself of any one food. Just go easy on some things that don't have a lot of nutrient value—such as candy, chips, and soda—and fill up on those things that do have a lot of nutrient value, such as whole grains, fruits, and vegetables.

Now let's look at a sample day of eating that models the recommendations of the pyramid.

Breakfast:
¾ cup orange juice
1 cup cheerios (they are whole grain)
½ cup low-fat milk

Lunch:
Turkey sandwich with lettuce, tomato, and mayonnaise on 2
    slices whole-wheat bread
½ cup carrot sticks
1 cup yogurt with 1 cup fresh blueberries

Snacks:
1 ounce string cheese with 6 crackers; 1 apple; ½ cup nuts

Dinner:
3 ounces grilled chicken
1 cup broccoli
½ cup rice
1 dinner roll with 1 teaspoon butter or margarine

This daily menu meets all the recommendations of the pyramid. You can add some "discretionary calories" if you like, by adding some baked chips with lunch and ice cream for dessert.

Dietary Reference Intakes

Between the Dietary Guidelines and MyPyramid, you have the basic tools you need to plan a healthy diet. However, you might be wondering exactly how much of each nutrient you need in your overall diet. The Dietary Reference Intakes or DRIs (there's an acronym for just about everything.) provide information on amounts of nutrients required in a healthy diet. The DRIs take into consideration more individual factors, such as age, gender, and whether or not a person is pregnant or breastfeeding. You can review the DRIs at the website for the Food and Nutrition Information Center.

http://fnic.usda.gov

There's an app for this. Check out the apps for your phone or mp3 player on the mypyramid.gov website. They are free to download and give some great tips on the food guide pyramid, exercise, and other healthy options for teens.

Find Your Fuel

CHAPTER

2

In Chapter 1, we said that your body gets its "fuel," or energy, from food. Let's spend a little time looking at the different sources of energy in the diet and how each source contributes to your nutritional health.

Energy for your body comes from calories in food. Basically, there are three food components that provide energy in the form of calories: carbohydrate, protein, and fat. You need all three of these components to stay healthy. Each one gives you different vitamins and minerals as well as other important nutrients.

CARBOHYDRATES

Your body's main source of energy (or calories) comes from carbohydrates. Carbohydrates are easily used by the body for energy, can be stored in the muscles for exercise, and provide lots of vitamins, minerals, and fiber. Each gram of carbohydrate provides 4 calories. You need from 45 to 65 percent of your calories from carbohydrate. The source of the carbohydrate is important. The best sources of carbohydrate from the pyramid are the grain group and fruits and vegetables. That is why they have the larger-sized strips on the pyramid; most of your carbohydrates should be from these groups. However, many Americans are getting too much carbohydrate from their "discretionary calories," especially from added sugars and sweetened beverages. Research is showing that a diet that is high in simple sugars may be linked with increased risk of developing Type 2 diabetes. Carbohydrates are definitely not all the same. Some are healthier than others. Let's look at the different kinds of carbohydrate.

Simple Carbohydrates

Simple carbohydrates are simple sugar units that your body can easily and quickly use for energy. Some simple carbohydrates are sugars, candies, sweetened gum, sweetened sodas, cookies, and cake.

Many foods have natural sources of sugar. For example, an apple or a glass of orange juice has the natural fruit sugar, fructose. Milk products contain the natural milk sugar, lactose. Natural sugars are not the sugars that you need to limit in your diet. Rather, it is added sugar that you need to be aware of. Excess intake of sugary foods has been linked with increased incidence of dental cavities. In addition, too much sugar can take the place of more nutritious foods in your diet. The best way to figure out if a food has sugar added is to look at the list of ingredients on the food label. Look for terms such as sucrose, corn syrup, and so on. When you see any of the following terms on a food label, it usually means that sugar has been added:

Sugar	Maple syrup
Sucrose	High-fructose corn syrup
Brown sugar	Chocolate
Confectioner's sugar	Dextrose
(powdered sugar)	Fructose
Corn syrup	Maltose
Honey	Lactose
Molasses	Glucose
Raw sugar	Fruit juice concentrate
Syrup	Invert sugar

Teens get a lot of added sugar from beverages. Take a look at the beverages listed in Table 2.1. Which beverage provides the most nutrition for the calories?

Table 2.1 Added Sugar in Common Beverages			
Food (8 ounces)	**Calories**	**Added Sugar (grams)**	**Other Nutients**
Milk, low-fat, 1% fat	95	0	Protein, calcium, vitamin D
Chocolate milk, 1% fat	142	12	Protein, calcium, vitamin D
Orange juice	102	0	Vitamin C, potassium
Sports drink*	57	14	Potassium, sodium
Cola*	93	24	None

*You should notice that the serving size here is 8 ounces, to be comparable to the size of a glass of milk. Most people drink at least a 12-ounce glass of soda or sports drinks. In fact, 20 ounces is the typical serving. So a 20-ounce bottle of soda really has about 60 grams of added sugar.

Complex Carbohydrates

Complex carbohydrates are sugar units that are linked together in chains. Also known as starches, complex carbohydrates must be broken down during digestion to provide your body with energy. Some examples of complex carbohydrates are pastas, whole grains, cereals, vegetables, and dried beans. Starchy vegetables include potatoes and corn.

The Dietary Guidelines recommend eating a variety of grains daily and making at least half of your grain choices be whole-grain foods. Whole grains provide complex carbohydrate and tend to have more nutrients and fiber than refined grains. Refined grains are carbohydrates that have been processed and have lost some of the nutrients in the processing. Eating plenty of whole grains may reduce your risk of heart disease.

Look for the word "whole" in the ingredient list on the food label, as in whole-wheat flour or whole-wheat bread. If the label lists just "wheat flour" or "enriched flour," it is probably not a source of whole grain. The following are some common terms on a label that indicate that whole grains are in the food:

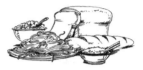

Whole-wheat bread	Whole-wheat pasta
Brown rice	Whole-grain corn
Whole-grain cereals	Oatmeal
Whole oats	Bulgur
Cracked wheat	Whole rye

The Dietary Guidelines also recommend eating a variety of fruits and vegetables every day. Fruits and vegetables are carbohydrate sources, too. As we said in Chapter 1, choose a variety of fresh vegetables and fruits. Think about color when choosing your fruits and vegetables. Lots of color usually means lots of nutrients.

What about Artificial Sweeteners?

Some people use artificial sweeteners, such as saccharin or aspartame. You can use these sweeteners like sugar by sprinkling them into your coffee or on your cereal. There are also products that contain artificial sweeteners, such as diet sodas, dietetic candies, and yogurt sweetened with aspartame. These products are usually labeled "sugar-free" because they contain artificial sweeteners instead of regular sugar. Artificial sweeteners are much sweeter than regular sugar, as much as 200 times sweeter, so you don't have to use very much of them to get the same amount of sweetness as you would with regular sugar. There are some newer sweeteners on the market that are considered "non-nutritive sweeteners" that are natural products with very few calories in a serving. The latest are sweeteners made from the stevia plant.

The leaves are naturally sweet, and the product made from the leaves has very few calories but compares to sugar in its sweetness.

Although people who use these products are often trying to reduce their calorie intake, no link between use of artificial sweeteners and weight loss has been found. Nonetheless, for people trying to reduce their intake of calories or simple carbohydrates, artificial sweeteners can be useful. People with diabetes often use these products because they have difficulty controlling their blood sugar.

The safety of some artificial sweeteners has been questioned. All products containing saccharin must be labeled with a warning to the public that it may cause cancer. It should be noted that the amount of saccharin consumed would have to be extraordinarily high to have such an effect. Some people with a disorder known as "PKU disease" cannot use aspartame. Others report side effects from aspartame, such as headaches, but these reports are rare.

If you use a lot of products that contain artificial sweeteners, you may want to limit your intake. For example, if you drink a lot of diet soda, substitute water or flavored seltzer water once in a while for a refreshing alternative.

PROTEIN

Protein is important for growth and tissue repair. Protein does provide energy in the form of calories, but only if other energy sources, such as carbohydrates, are not available. Like carbohydrate, protein provides about 4 calories for every gram. You don't need as much protein as carbohydrate, though. You need only about 15–20 percent of your daily calories from protein. Americans tend to get plenty of protein in their diets.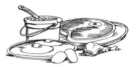

Protein is made up of building blocks called amino acids. Your body makes some amino acids. These are called *nonessential* amino acids. Other amino acids must come from the foods you eat. These are called *essential* amino

acids. A protein with all the essential amino acids is considered a
complete protein. Animal sources of protein, such as meat, milk, and
eggs, are complete proteins. A protein lacking one or more essential
amino acids is considered to be an incomplete protein. Plant sources
of protein don't contain all the essential amino acids that your body
needs and are therefore considered incomplete proteins. But eating a
variety of plant-based foods can provide you with all the essential
amino acids.

If you are a vegetarian, you may be getting all of your protein
from vegetable or plant sources. This does, however, require a certain
amount of planning and knowledge. See Chapter 6 for more information on plant sources of protein and vegetarianism. Table 2.2 shows
some common sources of protein and gives the amount (in grams) of
protein in a typical serving. You can see how easy it is to get the
amount you need.

Table 2.2 Common Sources of Protein	
Food Source	**Grams of Protein**
4 ounces grilled breast	34
4 ounces broiled lean steak	27
½ cup cottage cheese	14
1 cup cooked kidney beans	13
2 tablespoons peanut butter	8
6 ounces low-fat milk (1%)	7
4 ounces tofu	7
1 egg	6
4 ounces cooked pasta	6
2 slices whole-wheat bread	5

Extra protein in the diet isn't usually necessary. Contrary to popular belief, eating more protein won't give you more muscle. The only
way to make your muscles bigger is to exercise them. If you eat too
much protein, the extra amount not needed for growth and repair is

just extra calories. Extra calories, whether they are from carbohydrate, protein, or fat, get stored as body fat. See Chapter 8 on sports nutrition for more information on protein and muscles.

FAT: LIGHT, LOW-FAT, NONFAT

It seems that every time you turn around, someone is choosing a food that is lower in fat. Food companies keep coming out with new versions of their products that are lower in fat. People are always talking about how much fat is in food. Needless to say, fat has a pretty bad reputation.

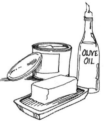

The truth is that fat actually plays some important roles in the body, and we can't live without it. First let's talk about what fat is and why we need it. Then we can look at ways to limit fat in the diet if it's necessary to do so.

The good news is this: we need fat. Fat on our bodies does several things for us:

- provides insulation to keep us warm
- protects our internal organs, such as the heart, lungs, and reproductive organs
- is a source of stored energy

Fat in the Diet

Fat in the diet has some important functions as well:

- It is an important source of essential fatty acids, such as omega-3 and omega 6-fatty acids (important in brain development, protection against heart disease, and eye health).
- It provides flavor to food.
- It gives us a sense of fullness in our stomachs.
- It helps carry certain vitamins around in the bloodstream (vitamins A, D, E, and K).

What we don't need is too much fat, either in our diet or on our bodies. Why not? Too much of certain kinds of fat in the diet can contribute to obesity (excess body fat) and can increase the risk of developing heart disease and certain kinds of cancer (see Table 2.3).

Table 2.3 Risks of Excess Fat in the Diet	
Obesity (excess fat of 30% over recommended weight for height)	Obese persons have a higher inci incidence of heart disease, stroke, diabetes, and some cancers. In addition, social pressure to be thin can make obesity difficult to handle emotionally.
Heart Disease	Excess dietary fat can cause elevated cholesterol in the blood as well as elevated levels of other blood fats that are known to be risk factors for heart disease.
Cancer	Excess dietary fat may increase risk of developing certain kinds of cancer, especially cancer of the breast, colon, esophagus, and prostate.

How much fat do we need? The Dietary Guidelines for Americans (see Chapter 1) recommend that teens choose a diet with about 25–35 percent of total calories coming from fat. So, if you're eating about 2,000 calories per day, you don't need more than 400–700 of those calories coming from fat. Because each gram of fat has 9 calories, that's between 44–78 grams of fat each day.

Keep in mind that these amounts are guidelines. On average, over the course of the week, your intake of fat should be between 25–35 percent of calories. There are days when you may have a little more than recommended and others days when you may have a little less. This is perfectly normal.

How much fat do I need?	
Daily Calorie Intake	**Grams of Fat Needed**
2,000 calories	55–78
2,500 calories	69–97
3,000 calories	83–116

To figure out how many calories you are getting from fat, it helps to know a little about where fat is in food.

How Do You Know How Much Fat Is in Food?

For the most part, if you follow the recommendations of the food guide pyramid, it's probably not necessary to count grams of fat or calories from fat. However, food labels do tell you how many grams of fat are in a serving of a particular food. See Chapter 12 for information on how to read a food label. If you know how many grams of fat are in the food, you can easily calculate calories from fat with a little math.

Each gram of fat has 9 calories. If a food item contains 10 grams of fat, it has 90 (10 grams × 9 calories/gram) calories from fat. Going a step further, to find the percentage of calories coming from fat, divide the calories from fat by the total calories in the food. If your food item has 360 calories in a serving and 90 calories from fat, the percentage of calories from fat is 90 ÷ 360 = .25, or 25 percent.

All Fats Are Not Created Equal

We've said that some fat is necessary in the diet. However, there are different types of fat, and some fats are better for you than others.

Two types of fats that are considered harmful to your health are saturated fats and trans fats. These types of fats have been shown to raise cholesterol in the blood and may cause heart disease.

Basically, fats can be either saturated or unsaturated. The saturation has to do with the chemical structure of the fat molecule. (Consult your chemistry teacher for more information on this one.) Saturated fats are usually hard or solid at room temperature. Foods high in saturated fat include fatty meats, the skin and fat on poultry, high-fat dairy products (cheese, whole milk, cream, butter, and full-fat ice cream), coconut oil, and lard.

Trans fats are usually human-made fats such as margarine. They are made when vegetable oils are chemically changed to make the oil solid at room temperature. This process is called hydrogenation. Trans fats or hydrogenated oils are found in many processed foods, baked goods, and snacks, as well as margarines.

Unsaturated fats tend to be liquid at room temperature. They include polyunsaturated fats, such as vegetable oils (corn oil, safflower oil), nuts, and some margarines. Unsaturated fats also include monounsaturated fats, such as the fat in olives, olive oil, avocados, and canola oil.

Too much fat, especially saturated fat, can increase your chances of developing heart disease later in life. Unsaturated fat does not tend to raise cholesterol levels. Replacing saturated fat in your diet with unsaturated fat can be a healthy choice. The Dietary Guidelines recommend that no more than 10 percent of your calories come from saturated fat and that you keep trans fat levels as low as possible. Food labels can help you figure out how much saturated fat and trans fat are in the food you eat.

For a given number of calories per day, there is a recommended number of grams of fat:

2,000 calories/day	21 grams of saturated fat/day
2,200 calories/day	24 grams of saturated fat/day
2,500 calories/day	27 grams of saturated fat/day
3,000 calories/day	33 grams of saturated fat/day

In addition, too much fat of any kind in your diet can contribute to too many overall calories in your diet. This can cause you to gain weight. Excessive weight gain has many health risks, as we discuss in Chapter 5.

What's Cholesterol?

Cholesterol is a waxy substance found in blood and in body cells. Surprisingly, we actually need cholesterol. We use it to make some hormones and vitamin D. However, your body can make all of its own cholesterol, so we really don't need to eat it. Nevertheless, cholesterol is found in many animal products such as meats, organ meats (e.g., liver), eggs, milk, butter, and shellfish. If you eat excessive amounts of these foods, your body may make more cholesterol than it needs.

Too much cholesterol in the blood may increase the risk of developing heart disease. The Dietary Guidelines suggest limiting cholesterol in the diet to 300 milligrams (mg)/day. You don't need to avoid cholesterol-containing foods; you just need to limit the amount you eat. See Table 2.4 for some common cholesterol-containing foods. You can see that just switching from whole milk to fat-free (skim) milk saves 22 mg of cholesterol. That is because the cholesterol is in the fat of the milk.

Table 2.4 Common Cholesterol-Containing Foods	
Food Item	Cholesterol (mg)
3 ounces beef liver	331
1 whole egg	212
4 ounces beef steak	76
3 small shrimp, boiled	32
8 ounces whole milk	31
½ cup vanilla ice cream	25
1 teaspoon butter	10
8 ounces fat-free (skim) milk	9

Choosing Lower-Fat Foods

If you think your diet may be too high in fat, there are some changes you can make.

- Keep the pyramid in mind as you choose your foods and emphasize eating more whole grains, fruit, and vegetables.
- Most whole grains, breads, pastas, and cereals are naturally low in fat.
- Fruits and vegetables have loads of great vitamins and fiber and very little fat.
- Choose lean meats, beans, and low-fat dairy products.
- Limit your intake of processed foods such as crackers, cookies, cakes, and other higher-fat snacks (this helps lower your trans fat intake as well).
- Go easy on the fast food.
- Check the label if you're unsure about the amount of fat in a particular food.

Here are some terms to look for: when cooking—broil, bake, grill, and roast instead of sauté or fry; when shopping—get familiar with the definitions of such terms as low-fat and lite. See Table 2.5 for definitions of some of these terms.

When eating out, look for broiled, baked, grilled, or roasted menu items. Ask for reduced-fat items or look for a "healthy heart symbol." Many restaurants offer menus that tell us exactly how many calories and fat are in their food items. This is really helpful, because there can be lots of hidden fat and calories when you are eating out. Choose low-fat salad dressings or have your dressing on the side so that you can limit the amount you use.

Looking for some good low-fat snack ideas? Table 2.6 gives you some delicious and low-fat options, including some of the recipes from Chapter 12.

LESS IS NOT ALWAYS BEST

Although it is beneficial to adopt the Dietary Guidelines for healthy eating and to keep fat calories between 25–35 percent of your total

Table 2.5 Common Food Label Terms Referring to Fat	
Label Term	**Definition**
Fat-free	A serving contains no or an insignificant amount of fat (less than 0.5 gram).
Low-fat	A serving contains no more than 3 grams of fat, no more than 1 gram of saturated fat.
Reduced-fat	The product has been changed to have 25 percent less fat than the original product or reference product.
Light (Lite)	The product has been changed to have at least 50 percent less fat than the original product or reference product.
Percentage fat-free	A product must be low-fat or fat-free, and the percentage must accurately reflect the amount of fat in 100 grams of the food.

calories, it is not good to restrict your fat intake too much. If you do, you may lose some of the benefits of fat, as mentioned earlier in the chapter. Fat provides flavor to food, so without fat your food may not taste as good. Fat leaves your stomach last, so it helps you feel full. Without enough fat, you may overeat as you try to fill that empty feeling in your stomach. In addition, research is indicating that some people are eating more calories even though they are eating less fat. Just because something is low in fat doesn't mean it has fewer calories. It also doesn't mean that you can eat more of a food because it is low in fat. You can easily gain weight on a low-fat diet. Many people do. It may be better to satisfy yourself with a moderate serving of real ice cream than to eat an entire half-gallon of nonfat frozen yogurt.

Think moderation, and choose the healthiest foods for you. Keeping the food guide pyramid in mind and balancing your choices really does work.

Table 2.6 Thirty Snacks with 30 Percent or Fewer Calories from Fat		
Food Item	**Calories**	**% Calories from Fat**
Popcorn(low-fat microwave), 3 cups	71	20%
Yogurt (low-fat),1 cup	240	10%
Breakfast bar, 1	136	15%
Fresh strawberries, 1 cup	70	0%
Graham crackers, 2	60	20%
1 ounce low-fat tortilla chips with ¼ cup salsa	130	6%
½ whole-wheat English muffin with 1 teaspoon strawberry jam	84	7%
Dairy Queen fudge bar	50	0%
½ cup vanilla pudding	160	28%
1 cup chocolate milk (1% fat)	158	14%
Fig Newtons, 2	111	18%
20 animal crackers	111	28%
Baked potato chips	110	14%
Colleen's Granola*	342	20%
1 medium banana	110	0%
1 cup Cheerios with ½ cup low-fat (1%) milk	133	19%
Pretzel twists	108	8%
Applesauce*	189	22%
Angel Devil Smoothie*	196	1%
Banana Shake*	321	13%
1 cup vegetable soup	72	24%
Mini popcorn cakes, 6	60	8%
½ whole-grain bagel with 2 teaspoons peanut butter	213	26%
8 baby carrots with Spinach Dip*	63	4%
Whole-wheat pretzels*	138	13%
*See Chapter 12		

There's an app for this!
There are lots of cool nutrition apps. You can get an app that has all quick nutrition tips, daily tips, complete nutrition information, and more. Test a few out.

KEY TERMS AND DEFINITIONS

calories: a measure of energy in food

simple carbohydrates: a sugar unit, such as glucose, that can be easily used by the body for energy

fructose: simple sugar or carbohydrate, found naturally in fruit

lactose: simple sugar or carbohydrate, found naturally in milk

complex carbohydrates: several sugar units linked together, e.g., starches

whole grains: grain containing all parts of the wheat kernel, including the bran

refined grains: grain that has had part of the wheat kernel removed in processing

nonessential amino acids: those amino acids that our bodies are able to make

essential amino acids: those amino acids that our bodies cannot make and that we must get from food

complete protein: protein source with all essential amino acids

incomplete protein: protein source missing one or more essential amino acids

saturated fat: type of fat in which as many hydrogens as possible are bound to the carbons; usually hard at room temperature

unsaturated fat: usually liquid at room temperature, with at least one carbon double bond

trans fat: naturally occurring and, more frequently, human-made fat—when liquid fat is made solid by adding hydrogen bonds

polyunsaturated fat: type of unsaturated fat with more than one carbon double bond

monounsaturated fat: type of unsaturated fat with one carbon double bond

cholesterol: waxy substance that is part of animal cells, found only in animal products

sauté: fry in a small amount of fat

Vitamins and Minerals

CHAPTER

3

Vitamins give you energy!
You need vitamin C to prevent colds!
Vitamin A clears up acne!

You've probably heard at least one of these claims and many others like them. With the plethora (a cool word, meaning "a whole lot") of information out there on vitamins, minerals, and supplements, it's a good idea to arm yourself with the most recent facts and decide how you can benefit. Does your diet have enough vitamins and minerals? Should you take supplements? Can supplements hurt you? Let's find out.

THE FACTS

Vitamins are nutrients that are found naturally in almost all foods. They are needed in small amounts, but they play many important roles in the body. Although vitamins do not provide energy in the form of calories, some vitamins are important in energy-producing reactions in the body. In other words, vitamins help your body make energy from the foods that you eat. Vitamins are usually classified as either water-soluble or fat-soluble.

The water-soluble vitamins, vitamin C and the B vitamins, dissolve in water. Our bodies cannot store them to use later. Any extra amounts that we eat are excreted in urine.

Fat-soluble vitamins dissolve in fat. They are stored in your liver and in body fat. The fat-soluble vitamins include vitamins A, D, E, and K.

Minerals are also nutrients that are found naturally in food. Some minerals, such as iron, are called trace minerals because we need them in such small amounts. Other minerals, like calcium, are major minerals needed in much larger quantities. Like vitamins, minerals perform many important functions in the body:

- They may help with the body's structure; for example, calcium in the diet helps build strong bones.
- They may help prevent disease; for example, iron in the diet can prevent anemia.
- They may even, in excess, contribute to a disease; for example, too much dietary sodium is linked with high blood pressure in some people.

Table 3.1 shows how each food group in the food guide pyramid provides many vitamins and minerals.

Table 3.1 Vitamins and Minerals in the Food Guide Pyramid	
Food Group	**Vitamins and Minerals**
Grains	B vitamins, iron, and copper
Vegetables	Folate, vitamins A, K, and C
Fruits	Vitamin C, vitamin A
Meats and beans	B vitamins, iron, zinc
Milk	Riboflavin (a B vitamin), vitamin D, calcium, and phosphorus
Fats and oils	Vitamins E, D, and A

You can see how easy it is to get all the vitamins and minerals that you need if you eat a variety of foods—in amounts consistent with the food guide pyramid recommendations. So, for most healthy teens, you can get the vitamins and minerals you need from the *food* you eat. Nevertheless, the store aisles are full of vitamin supplements aimed at improving your nutritional health (and possibly making a fair amount of money off you).

SUPPLEMENTS

Supplements are extra amounts of vitamins or minerals that are taken, usually in a pill form, to enhance your own diet. Sometimes people take supplements hoping that they will take the place of eating a healthy diet. In fact, many people take vitamin supplements as sort of "diet insurance" in case they aren't eating a healthy diet. Other people take supplements for a specific reason, such as to ward off a cold, lower their cholesterol, improve their heart health, etc.

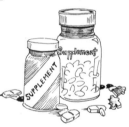

For starters, you should not take supplements without asking your doctor first. Vitamin and mineral supplements taken in large amounts (over 100 percent of the recommended amounts for that nutrient) can be harmful, even toxic (poisonous), to the body.

Nonetheless, when a person is not getting enough nutrition from diet alone, there are times when a vitamin or mineral supplement can be safe and effective. The most common and safest supplement is a multivitamin-mineral supplement. This supplement provides 100 percent of the RDI for individuals for most major vitamins and minerals. People who may benefit from supplements include the following:

- persons not eating the recommended number of servings from the food guide pyramid
- strict vegetarians (see Chapter 7 on vegetarianism for more information)

- people who cannot drink milk or other dairy products
- people on weight-loss diets
- pregnant or breast-feeding women
- women who are planning to become pregnant

There are lots of vitamins and minerals out there. We will highlight a few important ones that teens should know about.

Vitamin C

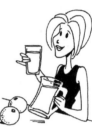

"Drink your orange juice so you won't get a cold." Vitamin C, also known as ascorbic acid, has several functions in the body. It helps repair body tissues and maintain the immune system. Your immune system helps you fight diseases and infections. In other words, vitamin C could help you avoid getting sick. Vitamin C is also an antioxidant. Antioxidants are substances that have been shown to help the body cells fight diseases such as cancer and heart disease. With all of the important jobs that vitamin C does, you can see why it's so important to get enough of this vitamin in your diet.

The recommended amount of vitamin C for most healthy people is 60 mg/day. Fortunately, if you like fruits and vegetables, it can be easy to get the recommended amount. Fruits, especially citrus fruits, such as oranges and lemons, contain lots of vitamin C. Vegetables, such as tomatoes, broccoli, and potatoes, are also great sources of vitamin C. Table 3.2 gives you an idea of how much vitamin C is in some common foods. A glass of orange juice gives you your full day's supply.

If you are not a fruit and vegetable eater, it is much harder to get enough vitamin C. The other food groups are not good sources of vitamin C. Everyone should eat at least 5 servings/day of fruits and vegetables. If you do this, you'll get enough vitamin C, as well as other vitamins and fiber.

Table 3.2 Good Sources of Vitamin C	
Most healthy teens need about 60 mg/day of Vitamin C	
1 8-ounce glass of orange juice	97 mg
1 cup strawberries	85 mg
1 medium kiwi fruit	75 mg
½ cup raw green peppers	45 mg
½ cup cooked broccoli	37 mg
1 baked potato	26 mg
1 raw tomato	24 mg

What about vitamin C supplements? Consuming extra vitamin C in the form of supplements is common in the United States. Vitamin C is often taken to ward off a cold or when you may be getting a cold. Even though the research is not definite on the real benefits of this practice, extra vitamin C is usually safe in amounts up to twice the RDI of 60 mg. Excessive vitamin C that is not needed by the body is excreted in the urine. Although vitamin C is generally not considered toxic, large amounts, over 1 gram (1,000 mg), can cause stomach upset and kidney or other problems.

Vitamin A

"Eat your carrots—they're good for your eyes." Vitamin A is found in carrots and is good for your eyes. It is very important in vision and has been shown to help prevent "night blindness" (difficulty seeing at night). Other functions of vitamin A include cell growth and maintenance of skin tissue. In addition, vitamin A, like vitamin C, is an antioxidant. As was previously stated, these substances help fight off cancerous cells.

Good sources of vitamin A in the diet include fruits and vegetables, especially those that are deep orange or dark green in color. Carrots, spinach, and cantaloupe are all great sources. Vitamin A also can be found in dairy products, liver, and egg yolks. Table 3.3 lists some good sources of vitamin A.

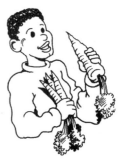

What about vitamin A supplements? Because vitamin A functions in maintaining skin, doctors often use it to treat acne and other skin conditions. Watch out, though. Excess amounts of a kind of vitamin A known as beta-carotene can turn your skin orange. High doses of vitamin A can even be toxic. That's because vitamin A is a fat-soluble vitamin, and we don't tend to get rid of it in the urine like we do with some water-soluble vitamins. Instead, the excess gets stored in the liver or body fat. Before you take extra vitamin A, by either putting it on your skin or taking a pill, ask your doctor. He or she can help you determine the benefits of vitamin A for you.

Table 3.3 Good Sources of Vitamin A	
Most healthy teens need between 800 and 1,000 µg RE* of vitamin A per day.	
1 medium baked sweet potato	2,488 µg RE
1 medium raw carrot	2,025 µg RE
1 cup cantaloupe pieces	516 µg RE
2 scrambled eggs	238 µg RE
½ cup cooked broccoli	174 µg RE
8 ounces low-fat milk	145 µg RE
1 cup canned peaches in juice	95 µg RE
*µg RE = microgram retinol equivalents, a measure of vitamin A activity.	

Calcium

Got milk? You'd better. You always hear that you should drink your milk. "It's good for your bones." It's true; milk is good for your bones. That's because it is such a great source of calcium.

Calcium is a mineral that is essential for proper bone formation and maintenance. Bones continue to form and grow until about age thirty. Unfortunately, teenagers, especially teenage girls, often do not get enough calcium. Insufficient calcium intake can result in osteoporosis later in life. Osteoporosis is a condition in which calcium is coming out of the bones, leaving holes in them. This makes the bones thin and brittle and more susceptible to breaking. People with osteoporosis can even end up with stooped posture and decreased height (yes, shrinking).

The best source of calcium in the diet comes from dairy products, such as milk, yogurt, and cheese. The calcium in dairy products is very well absorbed by the body. Some vegetables, such as spinach, contain natural calcium, too. However, the body is not very good at using some of these vegetable sources of calcium. Recently, new products have become available that have calcium added to them. These include calcium-fortified orange juice and cereals with added calcium. For people who don't drink much milk, these products might be a good addition to their diet.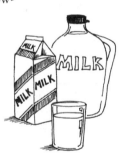

Teenagers need about 1,200 mg of calcium each day. You can get this by following the food guide pyramid recommendation of 3 servings from the milk group each day. Look at the labels on foods for information on the amount of calcium. Table 3.4 provides a list of good sources of calcium in the diet.

Girls who are concerned about calories and weight gain tend to drink less milk. Did you know that 1 cup of skim milk has fewer calories (and more vitamins and minerals) than a can of soda or a bag of chips? If you're not a milk drinker, try yogurt, cheese, or even ice cream. Here are a few tips for increasing your calcium intake with dairy foods:

- Try a smoothie.
- Have fat-free (skim) milk instead of soda at lunch.
- Snack on yogurt or frozen yogurt after school.
- Have cheese and crackers for a snack.
- Choose pudding and ice cream to satisfy your sweet tooth

Table 3.4 Good Sources of Calcium	
Most healthy teens need about 1,200 mg/day of calcium.	
1 cup regular or low-fat yogurt	400 mg
1 cup milk (fat-free, low-fat, or whole)	300 mg
8 ounces calcium-fortified orange juice	350 mg
1 ounce cheddar cheese	204 mg
1 ounce mozzarella cheese	147 mg
½ cup cooked spinach	142 mg
1 cup low-fat cottage cheese	138 mg
½ cup vanilla ice cream	85 mg

What about calcium supplements? If your calcium intake is consistently low, ask your doctor about taking calcium supplements. Calcium from food, however, is better absorbed than calcium from a pill. Try to increase your intake of calcium-rich foods—you'll get the added benefit of other nutrients at the same time.

Iron

A mineral of concern to teens, especially girls, is iron. Iron is part of hemoglobin in red blood cells. Hemoglobin helps carry oxygen to the cells. If you don't have enough iron in your diet, you could end up with "iron-deficiency anemia." This kind of anemia can make you feel tired all the time, short of breath, pale, and weak. Teenage girls tend to suffer from anemia more than boys do. This is due, in part, from the blood loss during menstruation in addition to poor eating habits.

Iron is found mostly in red meats. There is little absorbable iron in vegetable-based foods. That's why vegetarians need to be concerned about their iron intake. See Chapter 7 on vegetarianism for more information on this. You can increase your body's ability to absorb iron by including some vitamin C 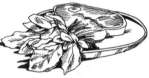 foods with your iron-containing foods at the same meal. For example, eating spaghetti sauce (lots of vitamin C-rich tomatoes) with meat in it (good source of iron) is a good way to up your iron intake. Another way to do this is to choose whole grains and enriched or fortified grains and cereals. Anything "fortified" with a nutrient has extra amounts of that nutrient. Table 3.5 gives you ideas on foods high in iron.

Table 3.5 Good Sources of Iron	
Most healthy teenage girls need about 15 m g/day of iron, and boys need about 10–12 mg/day.	
1 cup Total cereal (fortified with iron)	18.0 mg
1 cup Cheerios	4.5 mg
3½ ounces tenderloin steak	3.4 mg
1 broiled hamburger (about 3½ ounces cooked)	2.1 mg
2/3 cup raisins	1.8 mg
3½ ounces pork loin	1.0 mg
1 slice enriched wheat bread	1.0 mg

What about iron supplements? Supplemental iron may be prescribed by a physician if she or he finds that you are iron-deficient. Because iron can be toxic in high doses, you should not take iron supplements without a physician's approval first. You can take a multivitamin with iron as long as it provides no more than 100 percent of the RDI for iron. For a daily dose, the supplement should contain no more than 15 mg for girls and no more than 10 mg for boys. Ask your doctor and check the label.

VITAMINS FOR SPECIAL CONSIDERATION

Women and Folate

Folate, or folic acid, is a vitamin known to reduce the incidence of neural tube defects in infants when the mother takes it before she gets pregnant or early in the pregnancy. Neural tube defects are birth defects that result in incomplete closure of the spinal cord. This is a serious birth defect. It is important for all women of childbearing age to get enough folate in their diets.

Folate is found in leafy green vegetables, enriched or whole grains, liver, and legumes (beans). Grain products also are fortified with folate. So you can get folate when you eat fortified cereals and breads. Check food labels for folic acid information.

Sodium

Sodium is a mineral commonly eaten as part of sodium chloride, or salt. Americans tend to consume too much sodium in our diets, likely because we eat too many foods that are processed. Processed foods are foods that have been prepared and packaged with added sodium as a preservative or for enhancing the flavor. Processed foods are popular because of their convenience. They are usually quick and easy to prepare and serve. For example, packaged macaroni and cheese, prepared biscuit mix, frozen dinners, and canned soups are examples of processed foods. Usually the fresher the food is, the less sodium it contains.

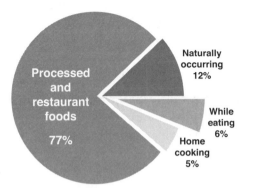

Figure 3.1 Most sodium comes from processed and restaurant foods.

We need only about 1 teaspoon of salt each day from all sources (sprinkled on food and in common processed foods such as crackers, cereals, chips, hot dogs, etc.). One teaspoon is about 2,300 mg/day. Too much sodium in the diet has been linked with hypertension, or high blood pressure. All Americans, including kids and teens, would benefit from reducing the amount of sodium that they eat. Most of our sodium comes from processed food, nearly 80 percent, and not from the salt shaker. (see Figure 3.1). Unfortunately, it is not that easy to figure out which foods are high in sodium. Some foods taste salty, such as chips and pickles, so you know they are high in sodium. Other foods have hidden sodium, such as some crackers, ketchup, and prepared spaghetti sauce. Here are a few tips to help you reduce your intake of sodium.

When you shop, do the following:*

- Buy fruits and vegetables for snacks instead of salty chips and salty crackers.
- Read food labels. Buy foods that say "reduced sodium," "low in sodium," "sodium-free," or "no salt added."

---

*Adapted from the Public Health Service, National Institutes of Health. National Heart, Lung, and Blood Institute.

- Choose fewer regular canned and processed foods such as sausage, bologna, pepperoni, salami, ham, canned or dried soups, pickles, and olives.

When you cook, do the following:

- Each day, cut back a little on the amount of salt you add to foods. You will soon get used to eating less salt.
- Use spices instead of salt. Season your food with herbs and spices, such as pepper, cumin, mint, or cilantro.
- Use garlic powder and onion powder instead of garlic salt and onion salt.
- Use less bouillon cubes, soy sauce, and ketchup.

When you are at the table, do the following:

- Take the salt shaker off the table.

VITAMIN D

In the past few years, vitamin D has gained more and more attention, with some experts even calling it a "wonder vitamin." We have known for years how important vitamin D is in bone formation, along with calcium. Now, the role of vitamin D is being looked at in relation to a healthy immune system. People who get enough vitamin D are able to fight off infections and prevent some diseases such as rheumatoid arthritis, certain cancers, and heart disease. No wonder people think vitamin D is a "wonder."

Unfortunately, many Americans (including teens) aren't getting enough vitamin D. It is found in fortified milk, fatty fishes, and oils (see Table 3.6). You also make Vitamin D when you are exposed to the sun. However, we know that too much sun exposure can increase your risk of developing skin cancer. And we know that teens aren't always drinking enough milk these days, so they may not be getting the vitamin D that they need. Teens need about 400 IUs of vitamin D every day. If you eat enough vitamin D-rich foods and get a few minutes of sun exposure each day, you probably don't need a vitamin

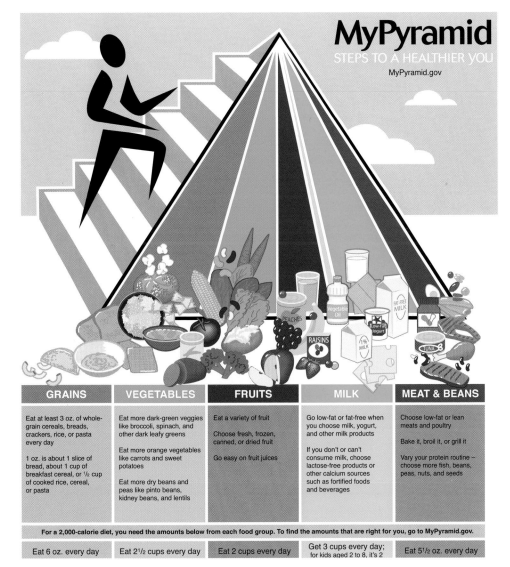

Figure 1.1. My Pyramid

D supplement. Your doctor can help you decide if you need a supplement. Vitamin D is stored in the body and can become toxic if you have too much, so you shouldn't take a supplement without asking your doctor about it first.

Table 3.6. Good Sources of Vitamin D		
Food	**Amount**	**IU**
Multivitamin (most brands)	Daily dose	400
Salmon, mackerel, sardines	3½-ounce serving	250–350
Shrimp	3½-ounce servings	200
Orange Juice (D-fortified)	8 ounces	100
Milk (any type, D-fortified)	8 ounces	100
Margarine (D-fortified)	1 tablespoon	60
Yogurt (D-fortified)	6–8 ounces	60
Egg	1	20

VEGETARIANS

Vitamin B-12 is important in nerve function in the body. A deficiency of B-12 can result in a type of anemia that causes nerve damage. Although deficiencies are rare, vegetarians may be at risk of B-12 deficiency. Vitamin B-12 is found only in animal products, such as beef and poultry. Vegetarians who do not eat any animal products should take supplements to meet their B-12 needs.

Another nutrient of concern to vegetarians is calcium. A vegetarian diet that does not include dairy products (i.e., total vegan) should include a calcium supplement. See Chapter 7 on vegetarianism for more information.

Table 3.7   Summary of Key Vitamins and Minerals

What is it?	Where do I find it?	What's good about it?	What about supplements?
Water-soluble vitamins			
Vitamin C, also known as ascorbic acid	Oranges, grapefruit, strawberries, broccoli	Helps fight off infection, helps heal wounds	Excess can cause stomach upset
Folic acid, also known as folate	Dark-green leafy vegetables, fortified grains, and breads legumes	Nerve function synthesis of genetic material. Important in prevention of neural tube birth defects	Take as part of pre-natal vitamin supplement during pregnancy
Niacin	Enriched grains, peanuts, meats	Energy metabolism	No real demonstrated benefit from taking as a supplement
Thiamin	Enriched grains, pork, legumes	Energy metabolism, nerve function	No real demonstrated benefit from taking as a supplement
Riboflavin	Milk, enriched grains	Energy and fat metabolism	No real demonstrated benefit from taking as a supplement
Vitamin B-6	Meats, whole grains, legumes	Protein , metabolism, red blood cell synthesis, immune system	Physician may recommend it for relief of premenstrual syndrome (PMS)

(continued on next page)

Table 3.7 Summary of Key Vitamins and Minerals			
What is it?	**Where do I find it?**	**What's good about it?**	**What about supplements?**
Vitamin B-12	Meats such as beef and poultry	Prevention of pernicious, anemia, nerve function	May be necessary for vegans and others not eating meat products
Fat-soluble vitamins Vitamin A, also known as beta-carotene, which is a form of vitamin A	Deep-orange and dark-green leafy vegetables and fruits such as cantaloupe, carrots, spinach, Also found in fortified margarine, butter, liver, egg yolks	Helps with vision, skin repair and maintenance	Excessive amounts can be toxic or, at the very least, can turn the skin orange
Vitamin D	Egg yolks, fortified margarine and, milk, sunlight	Bone maintenance	No real demonstrated benefit from taking supplement
Vitamin E	Vegetable oils, nuts	Cell membranes, antioxidant function	Not usually recommended as a supplement for teens
Minerals Calcium	Milk and dairy products, spinach, kale, fortified orange juice	Bone and teeth growth, repair, and maintenance, muscle contraction, blood clotting	May be necessary for someone unable to consume dairy products

(continued on next page)

Table 3.7   Summary of Key Vitamins and Minerals

What is it?	Where do I find it?	What's good about it?	What about supplements?
Sodium	Table salt, processed foods	Nerve transmission, regulation of fluid balance	Not usually recommended as a supplement for teens
Iron	Red meats, leafy greens, whole or enriched grains enriched grains	Red blood cell function, prevention of iron-deficiency anemia	Physician may prescribe it in cases of iron-deficiency anemia
Zinc	Meats, seafood, whole grains	Growth and development, immune system, wound healing	Not usually recommended as a supplement for teens

THE BOTTOM LINE

If you eat a healthy diet that is consistent with the portions in the food guide pyramid, you're probably getting enough vitamins and minerals. If you don't, you should first ask yourself "What can I do to improve my diet?" rather than "What supplements can I take to compensate for a poor diet?" In the end, if you choose to supplement your diet, a good way to start is to discuss it with your doctor and opt for a multivitamin and mineral supplement that provides 100 percent RDI for the nutrients included. See Table 3.7 for a summary of vitamins and minerals.

 There's an app for this. Several fun applications are available for your phone or mp3 player that give you updated information on vitamins and minerals, supplements, and more. Check them out—many are free.

KEY TERMS AND DEFINITIONS

water-soluble vitamins: vitamins that dissolve in water; examples are B vitamins and vitamin C

fat-soluble vitamins: vitamins that do not dissolve in water; examples are vitamins A, D, E, and K

trace minerals: minerals that our bodies need in small amounts, such as iron

major minerals: minerals that our bodies need in much larger quantities, such as calcium

antioxidants: substances that have been shown to help the body cells fight diseases such as cancer and heart disease

beta-carotene: a form of vitamin A found in dark-green or dark-orange fruits and vegetables

osteoporosis: a condition in which bones are weak and break easily because of loss of calcium

enriched: the addition of nutrients that are already present in foods to produce levels that meet specific government standards

fortified: the addition of nutrients to foods during processing (anything fortified with a nutrient has extra amounts of that nutrient)

Let's Move

This book is mostly about nutrition and healthy eating. After all, it is written by a couple of registered dietitians. But we would really be missing the boat if we didn't spend a little time talking about the importance of physical activity. Being healthy is about eating right and about including regular physical activity in your life. The two really do go hand in hand.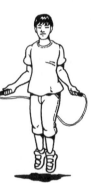

Unfortunately, kids and teens today are getting less physical activity than ever. It is probably no coincidence that our obesity rates are skyrocketing at the same time.

WHY DON'T TEENS GET ENOUGH PHYSICAL ACTIVITY?

There are loads of reasons for the lack of physical activity, most of which you teens are pretty familiar with already, right? I mean, you have to get up at the crack of dawn to go to school and maybe you have a job or clubs after school, you come home, you do homework, you chill out for awhile, and the day is over. Before you realize it, you haven't really expended a lot of energy even though you may feel tired. In addition, in today's high-tech world, we have dramatically reduced the amount of lifestyle exercise that all of us get, yet we still seem to be pretty busy. If you don't play a formal sport, club sport for your school, go to the gym, or work out on your own, it is highly probable that you aren't getting enough physical activity.

Okay, let's get right to it. First, we need to figure out how much physical activity you need and then decide if you are getting enough. Finally, we'll talk strategy—that is, how can you get more minutes of physical activity into your already busy day?

SO HOW MUCH ACTIVITY DO YOU NEED?

The Dietary Guidelines current recommendation is as follows:

- Teens should aim for at least 60 minutes of physical activity on most, preferably all, days of the week.

There are actually three types of physical activity that you should be participating in:

1. **Aerobic exercise:** This can include either moderate-intensity aerobic activity, such as brisk walking, or vigorous-intensity activity, such as running. Aerobic activity should make up most of your 60 or more minutes of physical activity each day. Be sure to include vigorous-intensity aerobic activity on at least 3 days per week.

   What Is Moderate-Intensity and Vigorous-Intensity Activity?*

   Moderate: While performing the physical activity, if your breathing and heart rate is noticeably faster, but you can still carry on a conversation, the activity is probably moderately intense. Examples include the following:
   - Walking briskly (a 15-minute mile)
   - Light yard work (raking or bagging leaves or using a lawn mower)

- Light snow shoveling
- Actively playing with your friends
- Biking at a casual pace

Vigorous: If your heart rate is increased substantially, and you are breathing too hard and fast to have a conversation, the activity is probably vigorous. Examples include the following:

- Jogging or running
- Swimming laps
- Rollerblading or inline skating at a brisk pace
- Cross-country skiing
- Most competitive sports (football, basketball, or soccer)
- Jumping rope

* From the Centers for Disease Control, *Physical Activity for a Healthy Weight*, www.cdc.gov/healthyweight/physical_activity/index.html.

2. **Muscle strengthening:** Include muscle-strengthening activities, such as gymnastics or push-ups, at least 3 days per week as part of your 60 or more minutes.

3. **Bone strengthening:** Include bone-strengthening activities, such as jumping rope or running, at least 3 days per week as part of your 60 or more minutes. We call these activities "bone-strengthening" because they involve placing weight on your bones. Exercise that involves some "pounding" on your bones, such as running and jumping, actually helps "pound" the calcium into your bones, making them stronger. Cool, huh?

If you play a sport and have practice 5 times each week, you are probably all set. In fact, you could jump ahead to the chapter on Sports Nutrition to read up on the best ways to fuel the athlete.

For the rest of you, this is the time to assess whether you are getting at least 60 minutes of activity each day. The good news is that this activity doesn't have to be all at once. You can get your 60 minutes in throughout the day. See Table 4.1 for an example of getting 60 minutes of physical activity and including different types of exercise in your day.

Table 4.1 How to Get 60 Minutes of Physical Activity				
Activity	Time	Aerobic	Muscle-strengthening	Bone-strengthening
Do sit-ups and push-ups in PE class	10 minutes		X	
Walk home from school at a brisk pace	10 minutes	X		X
Play basketball at the YMCA with friends	30 minutes	X		X
Walk dog after dinner	10 minutes	X		X
Total	60 minutes			

Having trouble getting motivated? Sometimes the day just gets away, and you haven't gotten around to being very active. It's okay to give yourself a break once in awhile. Just get right back to it the next day. If you find yourself having trouble getting motivated to stay with a routine or finding things to do, here are a few tips to help you.

TEN TIPS FOR STAYING MOTIVATED

1. Choose an activity you like. There is nothing worse than forcing yourself to do something that isn't fun. Physical activity is sup-

posed to be fun. Do something you enjoy. Maybe you hate to run but love to dance or play tennis.

2. Find a buddy, Exercise can sometimes be way more fun if you have someone to do it with. Set a schedule, meet at the corner to run or walk, play basketball with your buds, text each other to remind yourselves.

3. Consider joining a gym or the YMCA youth programs. There are lots of activities there for you to do and programs you might like to join.

4. Set a goal for yourself. Why not run your first 5K or bike a distance for a charity? Set a goal, create a schedule, and reward yourself when you succeed.

5. Do more of the little lifestyle things. Park further away from the entrance at the mall, take the stairs instead of the elevator, or hop off the bus one stop early.

6. Get a pedometer. Keep track of your steps, and set a daily goal to meet. There are lots of inexpensive pedometers available.

7. Download some apps. Wow—there are a ton of free apps for your phone or mp3 player. You can download a pedometer, a fitness tracker, and more. Check out the apps.

8. Try a fitness-oriented video game. Perhaps you are spending more time than you need playing video games. Your thumbs don't really need that much exercise. Try out one of the fitness video games, such as Nintendo Wii®. You can have fun playing Frisbee, tennis, and yoga while keeping track of your fitness goals. There is even a Body Mass Index or (BMI) tracker.

9. Get your family involved. Chances are everyone in your household could use some extra physical activity. Instead of renting a DVD, suggest some more active family time, such as hiking, rollerblading, biking, dancing, or a backyard game of baseball

10. Try something completely new. Maybe you are in a fitness rut—walking or running the same route or playing the same sport all

year. Try something else: Pilates, yoga, skiing, snowboarding, or one of the newer dances such as the Latin-inspired Zumba®.

Whatever you do, the key to physical activity is finding things you like to do and sticking with your routine. Daily physical activity will soon be as regular in your life as brushing your teeth.

 There's an app for this. Did you know you could download your own pedometer app? You can also download some really cool fitness apps to help you train for your first 5K or to learn Pilates.

Weight Management

One of the key messages in the Dietary Guidelines involves maintaining a healthy body weight as follows:

- To maintain body weight in a healthy range, balance the calories that you eat from food and beverages with the calories that you use being active.
- To prevent gradual weight gain over time, make small decreases in food and beverage calories and increase your physical activity.

Being overweight or being underweight can be harmful to your health. Being overweight can affect how you feel, physically and emotionally. You may have less energy to do the activities that you enjoy or even to participate in sports. As you get older, having excess body fat can increase your risk of developing heart disease, high blood pressure, diabetes, and other health problems.

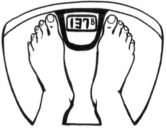

Being underweight can be harmful as well. You need a certain amount of body fat to protect your internal organs and to serve as an energy reserve. Underweight teens may not grow properly and tend to get sick more easily.

WHAT IS A HEALTHY WEIGHT?

Your healthy weight is the one that is just right for you. It may be quite different from your best friend's or your teammate's weight, even if they are the same height as you. But, you may wonder, shouldn't two people of the same height weigh about the same? Not necessarily. Your body type and frame size are inherited from your family. Other contributors to your weight include gender (males tend to weigh more than females) and muscle mass (muscle weighs more than fat).

It's important to find a weight for yourself that allows you to eat and enjoy healthy foods with your friends and to be active. The number on the scale may not be as important as how you feel and whether you can maintain a healthy active lifestyle at that weight.

OVERWEIGHT, OR OVERFAT?

Because we've just said that you could weigh more than is recommended for your height and still be at a healthy weight, let's use the term "overfat" instead of "overweight." Excess body fat is a better indicator of health than weight alone. A person can be within a so-called healthy weight range and still be overfat. He or she could be inactive, therefore having less muscle mass. Looking at body weight alone doesn't tell us if a weight is healthy for a person.

However, doctors and other health-care providers often use healthy weight and height tables, especially with growing children and teens, to track growth or look for potential problems. Significant changes in weight without accompanying changes in height could signal a problem. The tool most often used now to evaluate weight is the Body Mass Index, or BMI. This measurement uses an equation (yikes, math!), with height and weight being the variables.

The good news is that there is a BMI graph, so all you need to do is weigh yourself and have your height measured. Using the graph in Figure 5.1, find your BMI category. The BMI graph shows ranges that are considered healthy. Basically, the higher your BMI category is, the greater your risk may be for health problems such as heart disease and

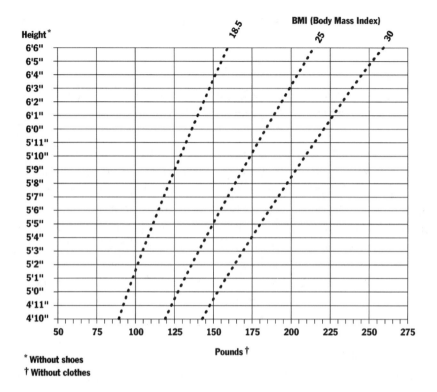

Figure 5.1 The Body Mass Index (BMI)

diabetes. You can also find a "BMI calculator" online at the Centers for Disease Control website. The website has some great information on healthy weight management: www.cdc.gov/healthyweight/.

BMI measures weight in relation to height. The BMI ranges shown in the preceding graph are for adults. They are not exact ranges of healthy and unhealthy weights. However, they show that health risk increases at higher levels of overweight and obesity. Even within the healthy BMI range, weight gains can carry health risks for adults.

Find your weight on the bottom of the graph. Go straight up from that point until you come to the line that matches your height. Then look to find your weight group.

- **If your BMI is less than 18.5,** it falls within the underweight range.
- **If your BMI is 18.5 to 24.9,** it falls within the normal or healthy weight range.
- **If your BMI is 25.0 to 29.9,** it falls within the overweight range.
- **If your BMI is 30.0 or higher,** it falls within the obese range.

If your BMI falls above the healthy weight, you may still be at a healthy weight for *you*, particularly if you have a lot of muscle mass or a large body frame. This is because muscle and bone weigh more than fat. You could, however, be at risk for weight-related problems if you have excess body fat. Unfortunately, body fat is hard to measure. It can only be accurately measured by a trained health professional. That's why most people simply use BMI as a general guide.

In addition, if you are overfat and have relatives who have heart disease or diabetes, if you smoke, or if you are not physically active, your chance of developing heart disease or diabetes increases.

If your BMI falls below the healthy weight, you could still be at a healthy weight for *you*, particularly if you have a very small frame. However, it is possible that you are underweight and at risk for related health problems, such as an eating disorder or impaired growth.

Once you've figured out a healthy weight for yourself, you need to work at maintaining that weight. By choosing healthy foods that fit in with the Dietary Guidelines and the food guide pyramid and balancing what you eat with plenty of physical activity, you should have no problem managing your weight. Keep in mind, though, that you are a growing teenager. You can and should expect your current weight, if it is within normal limits, to increase as you grow. Check your height and weight regularly (at least once per year) to see if you are within a healthy weight range for your height.

WEIGHT LOSS

Do you really need to lose weight? Find your BMI in Figure 5.1. Be realistic as you make this decision. If you are truly above the range for your height and you know there is room for improvement in the areas of exercise and diet, you may be ready to make some changes.

The best way to lose weight, if you need to, is to increase your activity level and choose a nutritious diet based on the Dietary Guidelines and the food guide pyramid. There are three things to pay attention to if you want to lose weight:

1. Get Your Engine Running (Increase Activity Level)

Increasing activity not only burns calories but also eventually increases your muscle mass. Muscle, or lean tissue, is a more active tissue than fat, which means that it actually requires more calories to maintain. People with more muscle can eat more. They even burn more calories standing still. Look for ways to increase your activity level whenever you can. You don't even need to start right off with a specific exercise program. Increase your lifestyle activities and you're likely to see results (see Table 4.1). 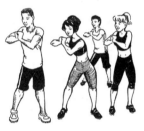 As you become more fit, you may want to incorporate a specific exercise into your life. See Appendix B for information on the number of calories burned during specific activities.

Unplug yourself. Did you know? A recent study by the Kaiser Family Foundation found that " 8–18 year-olds devote an average of 7 hours and 38 minutes (7:38) to using entertainment media across a typical day (more than 53 hours a week)."*

* Kaiser Family Foundation Report: Generation M2: Media in the Lives of 8- to 18-Year-Olds, January 2010.

Wow! So today's teens are spending over 7 hours each day "plugged in"—whether it is television, computers, video games, mp3 players, or texting on your cell phone. These kinds of activities are really encouraging you to be sedentary. In fact, obesity rates have increased dramatically in the past few decades among young people. Among the reasons is a lack of physical activity, accompanied by a large increase in sedentary activities, such as using computers, video games, texting, etc.

It may be time to take an honest look at yourself when it come to being too "plugged in." How many minutes or hours are you spending plugged in every day? Are you willing to reduce this a little bit? Consider taking a break every 15 minutes to go for an energizing walk. How about doing some activity-based video games, such as Wii Fit, dance video games, or other similar ones?

If you replaced 30 minutes of screen time with 30 minutes of walking, you could burn about an extra 150 calories/day. If you did this just 5 days/week, you could burn the equivalent of up to 11 pounds in one year. Take a look at Table 5.1 for some tips on increasing your daily activity level. It may be easier than you think!

2. Choose the Right Fuel (Watch What You Eat)

Now that your engine is running, let's look more closely at the fuel you use. It is really not a good idea to restrict calories when you are still a growing teenager. First of all, if you don't eat enough, you probably won't have the energy and stamina to do the activities that you enjoy. Second, you may end up compromising your growth; that is, you might not grow to your full height because you aren't eating enough calories to grow. Still, you should be following a diet that is in keeping with the Dietary Guidelines and the food guide pyramid. If you so, it's easier to get rid of those extra pounds. Ask yourself the following questions:

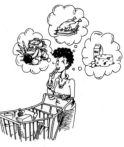

Do you eat at least 5 servings of fruits
and vegetables each day?   Y   N

Do you have at least 6 servings of whole
grains each day?   Y   N

Do you have at least 2 servings of low-fat
dairy products each day?   Y   N

Do you have 2 servings of lean meats,
dried beans, or nuts each day?   Y   N

Do you eat sparingly from the sweets,
fats, and oils group?   Y   N

**Table 5.1   Top Ten Tips to Increase Your Daily Activity Level
without Actually Exercising**

1. Hop off the bus a few stops early and hoof it.

2. Walk around the mall a zillion times (don't tell your parents we said to do this . . . it may cost them money).

3. Hide the remote (again, don't tell your parents we said this . . . although we bet they could use the activity, too).

4. Walk the dog. ✓

5. Walk your parents.

6. Leave the nearest parking spaces at the store for those who need them; park far away.

7. Dance.

8. Help clean the house or do yard work. (Okay, now you can tell your parents we said this.)

9. Play in the leaves, build a snowman (or rake the leaves and shovel the snow . . . Okay, we're parents here).

10. Take an energizing 10-minute homework break and walk around the block (or library or house).

If you answered *yes* to all of these questions, you are doing a great job. Keep it going. If you answered *no* to more than two of these questions, you've got some room for improvement. Start making those changes now. It's never too late to improve your eating habits, and the benefits far outweigh (no pun intended) the costs. You'll feel better, look better, and have more energy when you are at a healthy weight.

If you answered *yes* to most of those questions, but you are still putting on excess body fat, maybe you eat a healthy diet but you eat a little too much of it. See the next section for more on this.

3. Don't Overfuel

Believe it or not, it's possible to eat too much of a good thing. Paying more attention to portion sizes is crucial to weight loss and weight maintenance. The formula for weight loss is a simple one: too many calories in (in your mouth) and too few calories out (as in exercise or growth) = weight gain. It takes 3,500 extra calories to make 1 pound of body fat. If you eat just 100 extra calories each day (as in one 8-ounce glass of regular soda), that is 700 calories each week or a net gain of 10.4 pounds over the course of the year. This is just an example. Drinking a glass of soda every day won't make you gain weight, unless the calories it provides are consistently over and above what your body needs each day.

THE CALORIC BALANCE EQUATION*

When it comes to maintaining a healthy weight for a lifetime, the bottom line is this: **calories count.** Weight management is all about balance—balancing the number of calories that you consume with the number of calories that your body uses or burns off.

---

*From the Centers for Disease Control website,
www.cdc.gov/healthyweight/calories/index.html.

- A calorie is defined as a unit of energy supplied by food. A calorie is a calorie regardless of its source. Whether you're eating carbohydrates, fats, sugars, or proteins, all of them contain calories.
- Caloric balance is like a scale. To remain in balance and maintain your body weight, the calories consumed (from foods) must be balanced by the calories used (in normal body functions, daily activities, and exercise). For a closer look, check out Figure 5.1 and Table 5.2.

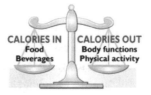

Figure 5.1   The Balancing Act

Table 5.2 Am I in Caloric Balance?	
If you are . . .	*Your caloric balance status is . . .*
Maintaining your weight	*In balance:* you are eating roughly the same number of calories that your body is using. Your weight will remain *stable*.
Gaining weight	*In caloric excess:* you are eating more calories than your body is using. You will store these extra calories as fat and you'll gain weight.
Losing weight	*In caloric deficit:* you are eating fewer calories than you are using. Your body is pulling from its fat storage cells for energy, so your weight is decreasing.

If you are maintaining your current body weight, you are in caloric balance. If you need to gain weight or to lose weight, you need to tip the balance scale in one direction or another to achieve your goal.

If you need to tip the balance scale in the direction of losing weight, keep in mind that it takes approximately 3,500 calories below your calorie needs to lose a pound of body fat. To lose about 1 to 2 pounds per week, you need to reduce your caloric intake by 500–1,000 calories per day.

BUT HOW MANY CALORIES DO I NEED?

Using the table from Appendix XXX ("Find Your Estimated Daily Calorie Needs"), we could say that the average teen female needs about 2,000 calories/day and the average teen male needs about 2,300 calories/day. But remember, calorie needs are different for every person depending on several individual factors. Your height, your weight, your age, your gender, and how much activity you do are all factors that affect how many calories you need each day.

There are some great websites with programs that let you enter your age, weight, activity level, and gender; then, the program tells you a recommended range of calories just for you. For example, the MyPyramid site is one that can do this.

Even though growing teens shouldn't be restricting calories, those with a BMI above the healthy weight range may need to look at their intake more closely. Perhaps they are consuming more calories than they need. Americans tend to eat very large portions of food. Advertisements are everywhere for mega-size, extra-large, and grande servings. Did you know that in the 1960s an average dinner plate was 8.5 inches and today it is 12 inches? Look carefully at the amount you eat. Don't fill up your plate. You may even want to use a smaller plate to help you decrease your portions. Did you know that it takes 20 minutes for our brain to tell our stomach that we're full? In that time, you can eat quite a bit of extra food and not realize that you are no longer hungry.

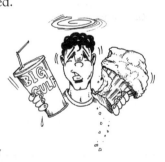

Maybe a simple hamburger will do instead of the double cheese-burger. Maybe a small order of fries is enough.

Pay attention to the amounts of foods you eat. You may even want to keep a food diary for a few days to see what you are actually eating. Check out food labels and see what a portion or serving size really is. That bag of chips may be meant for you to share with five of your best friends (i.e., servings per container = 6) instead of eating the whole thing yourself. If you find that you are still hungry after you've eaten, go back for seconds on the items that are nutritious for you first, such as fruits, vegetables, and whole grains.

THE SCOOP ON FAD DIETS

*Read the next paragraph and you'll lose weight—guaranteed...*Got your attention for a minute, didn't we? Now, you know that reading a paragraph in a book is not going to guarantee weight loss. Nonetheless, people try all sorts of crazy things to lose weight, none of which can guarantee anything.

It's almost impossible to open a magazine or enter a drugstore without being exposed to the latest and greatest way to lose weight fast. Now, come on, let's be realistic. If there really was a surefire, easy way to lose weight fast without diet or exercise, don't you think everyone would have done it by now? Why are there so many overweight people? Because losing weight is hard work. Harder still is keeping the weight off. It requires 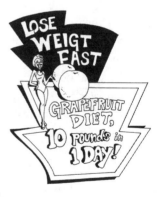 a change in attitude as well as a change in eating and exercise habits. Changing attitudes and habits is definitely hard to do.

Fad diets are just what they sound like: They're temporary, in and out of fashion, and don't offer a permanent solution. In some cases, fad diets can be truly dangerous to your health. How can you tell if a diet is a fad? Ask yourself the following questions when evaluating the latest craze in weight control.

1. Does it sound too good to be true? It probably is.
2. Does it promote weight loss of more than 1–2 pounds per week? Losing more than 2 pounds per week is usually associated with water and muscle loss, not fat loss.
3. Does it say you don't need any exercise? Forget it. Any good weight-control program must include exercise to maintain muscle mass and improve fitness.
4. Do you have to buy special food, pills, powders, or other products? You do? Who do you think stands to benefit the most? In the long run, it is the people selling the stuff who really benefit..

Table 5.3 summarizes various weight-loss schemes and why they don't work. Some even have serious side effects.

MEAL SKIPPING AND STARVING

Skipping meals is quite common, especially among girls, as a means to lose weight. Unfortunately, it doesn't work and may make the problem worse. Here's what happens: When you skip meals or starve yourself, your body gets confused. It really wants to eat and needs those calories for energy. So, when you do finally eat (and you will, eventually.), two things can happen. First, you may overeat at this meal, as your body demands the extra calories. Second, your body stores more calories as fat from this meal instead of burning them up for energy. The body is basically saying "Hey, I don't know when I'm going to get fed next, so I'm taking these calories and storing them up in case I need them later." That's not very efficient, and it won't help you lose weight in the long run. Your best bet is to feed your body healthy food at regular intervals so that it knows what to expect and can burn calories efficiently.

Long-term side effects of starving include hair loss, weakness, and constipation. In addition, starving causes dull hair (lacks luster),

Table 5.3	Weight-Loss Schemes: Why They Don't Work
Appetite suppressants (diet pills)	Often become ineffective after a few days or weeks. Many have serious side effects.
Diuretics/laxatives	Dangerous side effects. Temporary water loss, not fat loss. Do not teach you how to choose a healthy diet.
High-protein or low-carb diets	More water loss than fat loss. Can encourage a diet high in fat, saturated fat, and cholesterol, which is linked with higher risk of heart disease; extra protein can be strain on kidneys.
Crazy diets (grapefruit diet, cabbage soup diet, prayer diet, juice fasts, the fat-free diets, etc.)	Don't teach you how to eat from a variety of foods. Usually low in certain nutrients because iet is often missing or very low in one or more food groups.
Diet shakes, powders, etc.	Don't teach you how to eat from a variety of foods. Often low in fiber. Weight is usually regained.

cracked nails, paleness, and exhaustion. Doesn't sound too appealing, does it?

Table 5.4 summarizes the dos and don'ts for weight loss.

NEED TO PUT ON A FEW POUNDS?

What about weight gain? Some of you might feel that you're too skinny and want to put some weight on, perhaps in the form of muscle. Many of the same rules of weight loss also apply to weight gain. The only difference is that, in choosing foods from the food guide

Table 5.4   Summary of Dos and Don'ts for Weight Loss

Do plan your diet with the food guide pyramid and the Dietary Guidelines in mind.

Do exercise regularly.

Do limit fat in your diet.

Do snack, especially on foods with a lot of nutrients for fewer calories.

Do eat smaller portions of higher-calorie foods.

Don't try fad diets.

Don't take diet pills or diuretics.

Don't attempt very-low-calorie diets.

Don't starve yourself.

Don't skip meals.

pyramid, a person trying to gain weight is choosing from the maximum number of servings from each group instead of the minimum. For example, the grains group suggests 6–11 servings each day. A person trying to gain weight would try to eat closer to 11 servings instead of just 6 servings each day.

It is also important to do the following for weight gain:

1. Increase activity. Just because you don't want to lose weight doesn't mean you shouldn't exercise. As you gain weight, you want that weight to be in the form of lean tissue, not excess body fat. The way to build lean tissue is to exercise. Muscle and bone also weigh more than fat, so your scale will start to show the difference quicker, plus you will feel stronger and more energetic.

2. Watch what you eat. Being on a high-calorie diet doesn't mean eating lots of junk food. You need to eat plenty of nutritious food and use the food guide pyramid as your guide to portions and

quantities, choosing the maximum servings from each group. Choose nutrient-dense foods and include nutritious snacks in your meal plan.

SPECIAL CONSIDERATIONS IN WEIGHT MAINTENANCE

Adolescent Girls and Body Fat

Keep in mind that it is normal for adolescent girls to put on some body fat. It is their body's way of preparing for menstruation. In fact, you can't get or continue to get your period without a certain amount of body fat. That fat needs to be there to protect the uterus and allow for proper growth and development of a baby. If you restrict your calories too much and then notice that your period stops, you may well be losing too much body fat and are even on the verge of an eating disorder. (See Chapter 6 on eating disorders.)

Athletes: "Making Weight"

You want to wrestle in a certain weight class, but you weigh a little too much. So you vow to drop a few pounds before your match. Or you're on the cross-country team and someone tells you that if you lost a little weight before the meet, you might shave a little off your time.

Even though this doesn't sound like such a big deal, it is a big deal, with potentially life-threatening consequences. Whether you're a wrestler, runner, gymnast, or not even an athlete, losing weight rapidly can be extremely dangerous.

First, you're likely losing water, not fat. Why? Because it takes a calorie deficit of 3,500 calories to lose 1 pound of fat. Some athletes often try to lose several pounds in just days. It's virtually impossible to reduce intake and increase activity enough to lose only fat at that pace. The likelihood is that you are losing water and muscle—yes, muscle. Muscle loss means that the muscles get smaller and weaker.

Water loss can lead to dehydration, making you weak and dizzy. In the worst cases, dehydration can cause an elevation of body temperature as the body tries to cool itself. The end result can be death.

Table 5.5 lists the do's and don'ts for athletes who want to lose weight.

Accepting Your Body: "The Attitude Adjustment"

Often the way to change our appearance is to change the way we feel about our appearance. If I ask you to describe yourself, how would you answer?

If your answer involves your appearance—for example, I am blonde, blue-eyed, fat, thin, etc.—maybe you need to look more closely at yourself. Think in terms of your accomplishments, your hobbies, what kind of friend you are. These are ways to describe yourself, too. They are important indicators of how you feel about yourself.

Although losing weight may help you look better, try to focus on feeling better from the inside out. You may find that eating healthy foods and getting regular physical activity give you energy and an overall good feeling. It also helps to surround yourself with people who are supportive. Having family and friends who like you for who you are and support your new healthy lifestyle can be just as important as eating right and exercising.

Whatever size you are, be it thin or not-so-thin, tall or short, you need to remember that you as a person are not solely defined by your looks. Cultivate your mind, stay active and healthy, and learn to like yourself and others for who they really are.

 There's an app for this!

There are many helpful apps to get you started or motivated on your weight management plans. There are apps that count calories, track physical activity, give you daily motivational tips, provide nutrition information for many popular restaurants, and more. These can be terrific tools. Try a couple.

Table 5.5 Dos and Don'ts for Athletes Who Want to Lose Weight

Do consult with a registered dietitian and your doctor to determine the best and most realistic weight for you.

Do consult with your coach and let him or her know what weight you are comfortable with.

Do seek the help of another trusted adult if your coach or anyone else is pressuring you to lose weight.

Do eat a healthy, nutritious diet based on the Dietary Guidelines and food guide pyramid to maintain that weight.

Do strive to be a lean, mean fighting machine.

Don't try to lose large amounts of weight over a short time (no more than 1–2 pounds per week).

Don't try to sweat off weight unnaturally with saunas, overexertion, etc.

Don't let anyone try to convince you to do anything harmful to your body.

Don't keep calories too low. It harms your overall athletic performance.

Don't skip meals to lose weight. You usually end up overeating at the next meal, anyway. Plus, people who skip meals tend to have poorer nutrition than those who eat regularly.

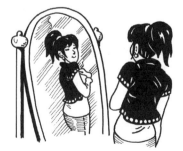

Eating Disorders

Or should this be called disordered eating? What does this mean? Eating is normal. Everybody does it. We need to eat regularly to keep our bodies going. So how in the world can eating become disordered? Does this mean "not in order" or "out of control"? Out of control is probably a good way to think of an eating disorder.

But first, what is normal eating? Normal eating is being able to eat when you are hungry and to continue eating until you are satisfied and then stop eating when you have had enough. It is being able to choose food you like and eat it. It is being able to get enough food and not just stop eating because you think you should.

There are several categories of eating disorders:

Anorexia Nervosa
Refusal to maintain even the lowest weight that is normal for age and height; distorted body image—thinking that you are fat even though you are underweight. In girls, it is often characterized by loss of menstruation.

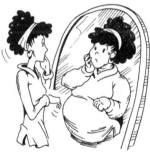

Bulimia Nervosa (often referred to as "bulimia")
Recurrent episodes of eating a great deal of food, eating out of control (at least 2 times per week), followed by some type of purging (method

of getting rid of the food so that weight is not gained). Purging is often done by vomiting, taking laxatives, exercising, or a combination.

Binge Eating Disorder (BED)

Episodes of eating great amounts of food but not purging. This behavior is often followed by feelings of guilt. Compulsive eating falls into this category. This is the most common of all eating disorders. Research indicates that 3.5 percent of females and 2 percent of men have this disorder at some time in their life.

Night Eating Syndrome

Eating 50 percent or more of the day's calories at nighttime, not being able to get to sleep or stay asleep, waking up during the night and eating, not eating in the morning. Considered a disorder if these symptoms occur for 3 months or longer. This is a real concern because of its association with obesity.

Subclinical Eating Disorders

This can be the early stage of one of the disorders listed previously. The female person may still be menstruating but has some of the symptoms of an eating disorder, such as anorexia nervosa, bulimia, or binge eating. Many individuals fall into this category in that they may occasionally binge, purge, or diet to lose weight. They may not have a full-fledged eating disorder yet, but they may be on the verge of developing one.

All eating disorders involve food and emotional problems that are associated with food. An eating disorder is a serious problem and needs to be addressed. Following are some behaviors you might watch for if you or someone has or is developing an eating disorder.

Common eating behaviors of people with anorexia nervosa are the following:

- Prolonged mealtimes; cutting food in very small pieces and moving it around the plate
- Secretive eating
- Avoidance of certain foods, such as red meat, fats, desserts, and breads
- Eating as little as possible during the day and saving eating for nighttime
- Choosing foods that have few calories so they are able to eat more (salads, low-fat yogurt, gum, sugar-free beverages)
- Eating as few as 300 to 1,000 calories per day
- Obsession with food

Common eating behaviors of persons with bulimia nervosa are the following:

- Eating low-fat foods
- Skipping meals and exhibiting irregular eating habits
- Limiting food choices
- Eating low-carbohydrate food when not bingeing
- Thinking of foods as good or bad
- Eating secretly
- Overexercising
- When bingeing, eating high-carbohydrate and high-fat foods; bingeing in private; usually bingeing in late afternoon or at night; feeling guilty when bingeing; often bingeing on convenience foods (not taking the time to prepare something)

If you or a friend is showing any of the eating behaviors listed previously, tell a parent, friend, teacher, school nurse—anyone who can assist in getting help for the person. Medical intervention is key.

CAUSES OF EATING DISORDERS

There are many theories as to why people develop an eating disorder.

- Culture. Society puts a great deal of pressure on us to be thin. We see this in our everyday life, in magazines, television, etc.

- Genetics. There may be some genetic predisposition to eating disorders as well: the makeup of your genes, your body itself.
- Physiological. Some scientists believe that there is a defect in some key chemical messengers in the brain that may contribute to the development or continuation of anorexia and bulimia. Compulsive eating may be the result of a defective mechanism in the brain as well. A message of satiety or fullness is not being sent.
- Psychological. People with eating disorders may have personal problems or family pressures. There may be negative early childhood experiences or psychological conflict in a person's life. Eating disorders often occur with other psychological disorders.

Whatever the reason, serious problems can result from eating disorders. Many people go throughout their life cycling from one type of eating disorder to another. It's important to get out of the loop as quickly as possible. The sooner that an eating disorder is identified, the more likely it is that this dangerous behavior will end.

WHO'S AT RISK?

Females

Teenage girls are the people we think of first when the term "eating disorders," especially anorexia and bulimia, is mentioned. And there is a high incidence in this group. It seems that girls who begin menstruating at an early age have more of a tendency toward these eating disorders than those who begin menstruating later. When a young woman begins to menstruate, many changes occur in her body. Her breasts develop; her hips increase in size. Eventually, she will be able to bear children. These changes can be very difficult for a young woman if they are not yet occurring in her friends. The early teenage years are a very stressful time. Young people want to be accepted, and if a young woman's body does not look like everyone else's, she may be concerned. Food is something that people feel they can control.

Athletes

Another group of people who develop eating disorders are athletes. Statistics show that 15–60 percent of athletes have episodes of eating disorders. Female athletes at risk may include gymnasts, dancers, and figure skaters. Female athletes need to be aware of what is termed the "female athlete triad": disordered eating, menstrual disturbance, and bone loss or osteoporosis (often leads to stress fractures).

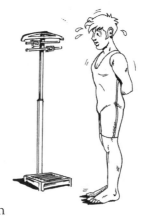

Male athletes at risk may include wrestlers, boxers, and football players. Many athletes need to maintain a certain weight so that they can either perform or participate in an activity. They may become involved in weight cutting for rapid weight loss. This is when an athlete severely restricts his or her food intake and depletes fluids by using steam rooms or saunas and by taking laxatives or diuretics to achieve a specific weight for competition.

Males

Although males account for only about 5–10 percent of anorexics and bulimics, they are still at risk. We all want to look good, and society does put lots of pressures on us. Young men have just as many difficult problems to face as young women do.

Other Groups

It's important to note that eating disorders can affect all socioeconomic and ethnic groups. In fact, recent research on young black women with binge eating disorders found that this group is at especially high risk for developing heart disease and diabetes.

COMMON CHARACTERISTICS OF PEOPLE WHO HAVE ANOREXIA OR BULIMIA

These are some common personal characteristics of people who have anorexia nervosa or bulimia:

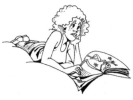

- Depression
- Low self-esteem, poor body image
- Self-destructive outlook, feeling as if they have done something wrong
- Difficult family relationships
- More frequent sickness because of low weight or poor nutrition
- Abnormal preoccupation with food and cooking
- Need to gain control over the area of life they feel they can control—eating
- Some obsessive-compulsive behavior, especially noted with bulimia nervosa

Persons with these characteristics may need professional help (e.g., counseling, psychotherapy) to get through a difficult time.

BEHAVIORS OF PEOPLE WITH EATING DISORDERS

Anorexia Nervosa

Anorexic behavior is more common in females. Often, these young women are overachievers and have perfectionist types of personalities. They are usually trying to gain approval of others. They are "people-pleasers." They view being thin as ideal. Usually, people with anorexic behavior are underweight and deprive themselves of food to maintain this low weight. They frequently obsess about food.

Bulimia Nervosa

People displaying bulimic behaviors may be overweight, underweight, or normal weight. Most bulimics are female and are usually older teens and young adults. They may show some obsessive-compulsive behavior. However, anyone may suffer from bulimic behavior. Most people with bulimia focus on weight control. Bulimics usually binge and may eat up to 20,000 calories at a time and then purge. They try to "undo" the bingeing behavior. Bulimics often are angry and are not able to express their emotions in an assertive way. They do not want to upset people. They turn inward and try to assert their independence with food and with the fact that they are able to control this behavior. Many bulimics are depressed or have a history of depression in their family. Some bulimics abuse alcohol or drugs as well as food.

Often, bulimia nervosa and overeating are grouped together. The reason for this is that both disorders involve compulsive eating. Both groups are usually obsessed with food. Whereas normal eating involves eating that is followed by a feeling of fullness or satiety, with overeating, fullness is ignored or perhaps does not occur. With both disorders, there is difficulty controlling eating behavior. There is an addiction to food. Once these people begin eating, they are unable to stop.

COMPULSIVE EATING

Compulsive eating often begins in early childhood. For many people, food may be a source of comfort. Some people overeat because it makes them feel good. One of the negative side effects of compulsive eating is obesity. Being obese puts one at risk for many health problems. Many people also feel that there are social problems associated with obesity, such as feelings of being "left out." This leads to decreased social acceptance and even to fewer opportunities for career growth later in life. Other psychological problems may develop for the compulsive eater as well.

MEDICAL PROBLEMS AND TREATMENT

Needless to say, eating disorders are serious and cannot be ignored. Table 6.1 lists some medical problems that might occur with anorexia and bulimia.

**Table 6.1   Medical Problems That Might Occur
with Anorexia Nervosa and Bulimia Nervosa**

Anorexia Nervosa

Death rates of 10%
Heart disease: most common medical cause of death

- Slow heart rhythm
- Low blood pressure
- Decreased size of heart
- Increased cholesterol levels

Kidney problems
Electrolyte imbalance as a result of starvation and decrease in fluid intake
Low levels of reproductive hormones
Increased levels of stress hormones
Decrease in growth in young adult
Irregular or absent menstruation
Bone and tooth deterioration: may lead to osteoporosis
Anemia due to poor nutrition

Bulimia Nervosa

Tooth erosion and cavities
Gum problems
Acute stomach distress
Irritation of throat and esophagus
Tendency toward compulsive behaviors, such as alcoholism and drug abuse
Electrolyte imbalance as a result of induced vomiting and diarrhea
Heart problems

Eating disorders are often more about the mind than about the food itself. An individual with an eating disorder often feels angry and upset and even guilty. But it is also very scary to look at the physiological problems caused by withholding food. Therefore it is vital to get treatment—and the sooner the better. There is a much better chance that eating-disordered behavior can be stopped if help begins early. Treatment from various health-care professionals is a must. Usually, a medical doctor, a psychologist or social worker, and a dietitian work as a team to help people with eating disorders. It is also important that the person's family be involved in his or her therapy. If you have a friend, a sister, or a brother with an eating disorder, be supportive and share your concern with them. Don't let them keep it a secret. Tell someone who can help him or her to get the proper medical advice. Be a friend!

ACCEPTING YOUR BODY

Ten Facts to Consider on Body Image*

1. The average model today is 25 percent thinner than the national average weight and actually only represents 5 percent of females in the country.
2. Almost 54 percent of young girls in the United States and women aged 12–23 years are unhappy with their bodies.
3. One third of high-school students think that they are overweight, even when they are not.
4. Eighty percent of women who answered a People Magazine survey responded that images of women on television and in the movies make them feel insecure.
5. One-half of fourth-grade girls are on a diet.
6. The average U.S. woman is 5'4" and weighs 140 pounds. In contrast, the average U.S. model is 5'11" and weighs 117 pounds.
7. Fifty-one percent of 9- and 10-year-old girls stated that they felt better about themselves when they were adhering to a diet.
8. A study found that adolescent girls were more fearful of gaining weight than of cancer, nuclear war, or losing their parents.
9. Some of the pictures of the models in magazines do not really exist. The pictures are computer-modified compilations of different body parts.
10. Eating disorders have the highest mortality rate of all mental illnesses. The mortality (death) rate for eating disorders is approximately 18 percent in 20-year studies and 20 percent in 30-year follow-up studies.

---

* Eating Disorder Foundation, American Association of Obstetrics and Gynecology

The road to recovery from an eating disorder can be a bumpy one. It is important for a person with an eating disorder or on the verge of developing one to be surrounded with people who are supportive. Having family and friends who like you for who you are and are supportive of your new healthy lifestyle can be just as important as eating right and exercising.

WHERE TO GET HELP FOR AN EATING DISORDER

If you or a friend has an eating disorder, find a trusted adult to confide in—a parent, teacher, school nurse, or coach. There are many organizations and books devoted to eating disorders. Check out the following websites and self-help groups listed. The sooner that a person with an eating disorder gets help, the better the chances will be for a full recovery.

WEBSITES AND ORGANIZATIONS

National Association of Anorexia Nervosa and Associated Disorders: www.anad.org/; 1-847-831-3438

The Eating Disorder Foundation: www.eatingdisorderfoundation.org/; 1-303-322-3373

National Eating Disorders Association: www.nationaleatingdisorders.org/; 206-382-3587

KEY TERMS AND DEFINITIONS

Binge eating: eating large amounts of food over a short time, accompanied by feelings of guilt at not being able to stop

Purging: means of emptying the body of what has been eaten, often by self-induced vomiting, taking medication that induces vomiting, taking laxatives, or exercising excessively

Laxative: medication that increases the movement of digested food through the bowel. The body may absorb fewer calories, and excess water may be lost.

Diuretic: medication that increases urination and promotes water loss of the body

Emetic: medication that induces vomiting

Obsessions: recurrent or persistent mental images, thoughts, or ideas

Compulsive behavior: repetitive, rigid, or self-prescribed routines

Osteoporosis: a condition in which bones are weak and break easily because of loss of calcium

Vegetarianism

CHAPTER
7

It seems, for some people, that being a vegetarian is "in" nowadays. But what actually is a vegetarian? This word has different meanings to different people. It's like choosing a fuel for your car. You can use different fuels, but you need to be sure that your car can handle the one you've chosen. Let's look at some of the possibilities.

WHAT IS A VEGETARIAN?

Technically, a vegetarian is someone who eats vegetables. Usually, a vegetarian is also someone who chooses not to eat meat or meat products. However, there are really several different kinds of vegetarians.

For example, a *vegan* is a vegetarian who doesn't eat any meat or meat products. A *lacto-ovo vegetarian* doesn't eat the flesh of animals but consumes milk and eggs. There's even a *fruitarian*, although this type of diet seems pretty extreme. A strict fruitarian eats primarily fruits, nuts, honey, and vegetable oils. This could lead to serious nutrient deficiencies.

Table 7.1 lists the different types of vegetarians and the foods they do or don't eat.

WHY BE A VEGETARIAN?

Just as there are many kinds of vegetarianism, there are many reasons why people choose to be vegetarian.

Table 7.1 Different Types of Vegetarians	
Vegan	Eats no animal or fish products at all, including dairy products, eggs, and honey.
Lacto vegetarian	Eats no meat, fish, or eggs but eats dairy products, such as milk, cheese, and ice cream.
Lacto-ovo-vegetarian	Eats no meat, poultry, or fish but eats dairy products and eggs.
Semi-vegetarian or flexitarian	Usually eats no red meat but generally eats dairy products, eggs, fish, and poultry. Some may just eat fish. Not true vegetarians.
Fruitarian	Eats only plant foods and some legumes and is concerned with the way the food products are harvested so that the plant continues to live.

- Taste. Some people just don't like the taste of meat, so they choose not to eat it.
- Ethics. Ethics comes into play for some people. Ethics, according to a definition in Webster's Dictionary, is "the discipline dealing with what is good and bad and with moral duty and obligation." Some vegetarians think that eating something that has to be killed so that it becomes food for people is just gruesome. Others think it is terrible to eat anything that comes from something living, even milk from a cow or an egg from a chicken. These decisions are totally personal, and each individual needs to make decisions on his or her own.
- Religion. Some people decide to be a vegetarian for religious reasons. Certain religions restrict meats or meat products.
- Health. People may choose vegetarianism for health reasons or weight control. They think that vegetarian eating is usually lower in fat and calories and is better for them. This may be true, but only if they are choosing a healthy vegetarian diet. Just as there

are poor choices in a nonvegetarian diet, there can be poor choices in a vegetarian diet.

- Environment. Many believe that they are being responsible citizens by not eating meat. The United Nations published a report in 2006 that stated that livestock agriculture is a major contributor to production of green house gases, which impact global warming. So eating meat and dairy products do have an impact.

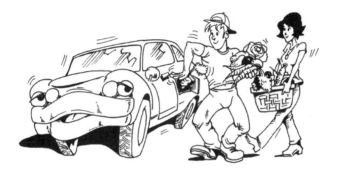

THE VEGETARIAN FOOD PYRAMID

Being a vegetarian isn't just about avoiding meat. You can end up a "Twinkie vegetarian," that is, someone who doesn't eat meat but fills her or his diet with foods of little nutritional value. Remember the food guide pyramid from Chapter 1? Well, there's a pyramid for vegetarians, too (Figure 7.1). It provides amounts and servings of foods so that vegetarians can get all the nutrition they need.

The American Dietetic Association published a *Position Paper on Vegetarian Diets* in 2009. The research indicates that people who follow a vegetarian diet have lower cholesterol, lower risk of heart disease, lower blood pressure, and less risk of type 2 diabetes. In addition, vegetarians usually have a lower BMI and lower cancer rates. This is because vegetarian diets generally are lower in saturated fat and cholesterol and are higher in dietary fiber and other nutrients that may not be as high in a meat-based diet. It's important to remember that vegetarians still need to have a nutritionally balanced

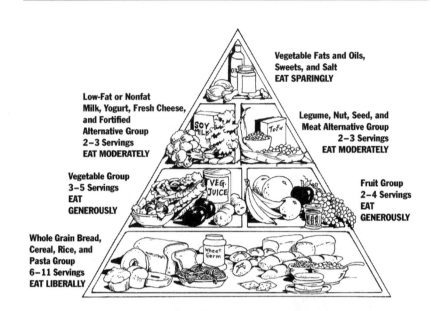

Figure 7.1 Vegetarian Food Pyramid

diet. Also, people who are vegetarians may be more physically active and may not smoke or drink alcohol—so vegetarians may have an overall healthy lifestyle that most likely contributes to decreasing their risk for the diseases mentioned.

It seems that the key is being health conscious. So choose what you want to be for the correct reasons. You can be a vegetarian and eat healthfully throughout your life.

NUTRIENTS OF SPECIAL CONCERN TO VEGETARIANS

Everything sounds great so far, so is there anything bad about being a vegetarian? Well, if you decide you want to give this lifestyle a try, there are a few things to think about. It's a good idea to be aware of a few nutrients that can be of special concern to vegetarians.

Protein

As a vegetarian, you can meet your intake for protein, but remember to eat enough calories for your weight (see Chapter 5 on weight management for calorie needs). If you are a vegan (i.e., eat no animal protein), you are able to get adequate protein in a variety of fruits, vegetables, and grains. Variety is really the key. There are eight essential amino acids, and if you are able to eat all of these throughout the day, you should be able to meet your protein needs. A complete protein has all the essential amino acids. When we combine these, we call them *complementary* proteins.

Vegetable protein usually does not have all the essential amino acids, so we call it an *incomplete* protein. However, although one vegetable or grain may be missing an amino acid, another may have it. If you eat the foods during the day, you can get all the essential amino acids. This is called "complementing proteins." You combine proteins from different sources so that all of the essential amino acids are obtained. You do not have to combine these items at the same meal, but you need to be aware over the course of a day that you have eaten a good combination of food items. Eating a variety of plant-based foods can provide you with all the essential amino acids. There are several good resources containing information on the amino acid content of foods. Check out the Resource section of this book under "Vegetarianism."

If you're not a vegan and eat eggs and milk, you don't need to worry about complementing proteins because eggs, milk, yogurt, ice cream, etc., are great complete protein sources. If you are a vegan, foods that are good sources of protein include legumes (beans and peas), grains, seeds, and nuts. Here are some common vegetarian food combinations. Each gives you a complete protein.

Rice and beans
Corn tortillas and black beans
Hummus and pita bread
Peanut butter on whole grain bread

Omega-3 (DHA) fatty acids

There are two fatty acids (omega-3 and omega-6 fatty acids) that are essential to our diet. They are essential for us to eat because our bodies cannot make them. Vegetarian diets are usually rich in omega-6 fatty acids but are low in omega-3. If you are a vegan, you need to get some DHA. Luckily, there are DHA supplements available, and soy milk and many breakfast bars are fortified with DHA. Make sure to check out the labels.

Iron

This sounds a little strange: vegetarians actually have higher iron intakes than people who eat animal products. But, compared to the iron in meat, the iron in plants is not as well absorbed by the body. That means that you need to eat a little more iron than nonvegetarians do. In other words, make sure you eat plenty of foods high in iron. Many breads and cereals are enriched with iron, so including enriched grains in your diet helps increase iron intake. Other plant sources of iron include the following:

Legumes (beans or peas)
Spinach
Beet greens
Bulgur
Raisins
Prune juice
Dried fruits

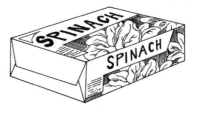

It also helps to consume foods containing vitamin C when you're eating foods that contain iron. Vitamin C helps the body absorb iron. So have some orange juice, a grapefruit, broccoli, or tomatoes with your spinach or enriched grains.

Finally, you can increase your iron by using cast iron pans when you cook. So ask a parent or grandparent if they have any of those put away somewhere, and get cooking.

Calcium

The teen years are when you are determining the density of your bones (how hard and strong they are). At your age, it's really important to have enough calcium because it contributes to that density. If you are a lacto-ovo vegetarian, you're probably getting enough calcium because you are drinking milk, eating yogurt, ice cream, and other foods that are high in calcium (see Chapter 3 on vitamins and minerals for foods high in calcium).

But, if you're a vegan, your intake of calcium is likely to be low. Try to include at least three sources of calcium each day. You may also want to ask your doctor about a calcium supplement. A few plant sources of calcium include the following:

Leafy green vegetables, such as collard greens, turnip greens, kale
Broccoli
Tofu prepared with calcium
Fortified soy milk
Calcium-fortified breads and waffles
Calcium-fortified orange juice

Vitamin B-12

You need vitamin B-12 for nerve function. Although plant food has some B-12, it is not a good source. It is recommended that vegetarians, and vegans in particular, take a B-12 supplement or make sure that they eat foods that are fortified with B-12, that is, have B-12 added to them to help meet these requirements. There are vegetarian products, such as cereals, that have been fortified with B-12.

Vitamin D

Vitamin D works with calcium to keep your bones strong. It's hard to get vitamin D in your diet unless you use fortified products. The one fortified product most of us get this in is milk. If you're a vegan,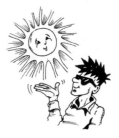

this may be a problem. You may need another source; try fortified soy milk. Or what about getting a little sunshine? Just 5 to 15 minutes of sun exposure a day is said to provide enough vitamin D.

Zinc

Zinc is vital to growth and development. The best source of zinc is red meat. Plant sources of zinc are not very well absorbed. Some good plant sources of zinc are the following:

Whole grains
Legumes (beans and peas)
Nuts
Tofu

If you don't think you're getting enough zinc by what you're eating, you should talk to your doctor about taking a multivitamin and mineral supplement that contains zinc.

VEGETARIAN RECIPE SUBSTITUTIONS

There are many excellent vegetarian recipes. We've included some in this book as well as provided resources so that you can find more recipes. If you like to cook, you may need to substitute some ingredients in your own recipes to make them vegetarian. Here are some ideas for when you cook with traditional recipes that use eggs, milk and dairy products, and meats. Try these substitutes:

Egg Replacers (these are used to bind or hold things together)
For 1 egg

- 1 banana
- ¼ cup mashed potatoes
- 2 tablespoons of cornstarch, potato starch, or arrowroot
- ¼ cup applesauce or pureed prunes
- ¼ cup tofu for 1 egg (blend tofu with liquid ingredients until smooth before adding to dry ingredients)
- Commercial "egg replacer"

Milk and Dairy Substitutes

- Soy milk
- Soy margarine
- Soy yogurt
- Nut milks (make them by blending nuts with water and strain)
- Rice milk (blend cooked rice with water)

Meat Substitutes

- Tempeh (cultured soybeans with a chewy texture)
- Tofu (if you freeze and thaw it, it gets a meaty texture)
- Wheat gluten or seitan (made from wheat and has a meatlike texture; is available in health food and Asian markets)
- Vegetarian burgers (often found in the frozen food section of the store)

BEING A VEGETARIAN AND EATING OUT

Although only 3 percent of Americans are vegetarians, many people are experimenting with this type of diet, and, as a result, it is easier to find vegetarian options when you are eating out. Even fast-food restaurants have options available. Did you know that Burger King has a flame-broiled veggie burger? Baskin & Robbins has dairy-free and gelatin-free ices and sorbet, and Chipotle serves a vegetarian fajita burrito.

It is easier to eat out if you are a lacto-ovo vegetarian than if you are a vegan. Try to include a milk, yogurt, or cheese source, some whole grains, and fruits or vegetables in your meal. At school, this amounts to a yogurt, a piece of fruit, a bagel, and any other items you need to round out the meal and have it be enough food for you. If you are a vegan, you need to do some advance planning and may be bringing your lunch from home. You will probably find that more and more schools are offering some options as vegetarian foods become more popular. Some school cafeterias offer hummus; others might have veggie burgers, a Portobello burger sandwich, or a vegan pita pocket. You can ask the food service director in your school if and when vegetarian dishes are offered.

In a restaurant, the choices are similar. You can usually get milk, bread, and salad at most restaurants, even fast-food restaurants. You can also often find baked potatoes or rice and ask for cheese to put on them. Meatless pizza or bean burritos can be great choices and are readily available. What you want to avoid is choosing the lower-nutrient dense foods just because they don't have meat in them. A cola and a large order of fries may be vegetarian, but it's not a nutritious meal.

BEING A VEGETARIAN WHEN YOUR FAMILY IS NOT

Your parents may have a difficult time adjusting to your vegetarianism if they are not vegetarians themselves. You can help them support your vegetarianism by being involved in menu planning and demonstrating your knowledge of healthy food. Offer to accompany your parents on a grocery trip or even offer to do the shopping on occasion. Familiarize them with the foods you are eating. Have a taste test. They may actually like some of these items.

Lots of everyday dishes such as pasta, pizza, tacos, and salads can be prepared to serve both vegetarians and nonvegetarians. Reassure your family that you don't expect them to short-order cook for you. If everyone stays flexible, creative, and respectful of each other's wishes, your vegetarianism shouldn't create a problem in your family.

SUMMING UP VEGETARIANISM

It really doesn't matter why you choose vegetarianism. You can always change your mind at any time or become a different kind of vegetarian than the one you are now. Regardless of your reasons, being a vegetarian can be a tough path to follow. To do it healthfully, you need to be knowledgeable about food and willing to spend some time learning about vegetarianism. It helps if you really enjoy planning and preparing meals. There are many quick and easy vegetarian dishes to prepare and many more vegetarian products available in the grocery stores than there were just a few years ago. So, if being a vegetarian is what you choose, go for it. Use the fuel that's best for you.

There's an app for this. There are several different apps available that relate to vegetarianism. For example, you can download an app on organic foods, fruits, and veggies. You can download an app that tells you nutrition information at your favorite restaurants so you can see ahead of time whether or not they have good vegetarian choices for you.

KEY TERMS AND DEFINITIONS

Vegan: someone who eats no animal or fish products at all, including dairy products, eggs, and honey

Lacto vegetarian: someone who eats no meat, fish, or eggs but eats dairy products, such as milk, cheese, and ice cream

Lacto-ovo-vegetarian: someone who eats no meat, poultry, or fish but eats dairy products and eggs

Semi-vegetarian: someone who eats no red meat but generally eats dairy and egg products, fish, and fowl (poultry)

Fruitarian: someone who eats only plant foods and some legumes and is concerned with the way the food products are harvested so that the plant continues to live

Complete protein: a food source of protein that contains all essential amino acids

Incomplete protein: a food source of protein that is missing one or more of the essential amino acids

Enriched: the addition of nutrients that are already present in foods to levels that meet specific government standards

Fortified: the addition of nutrients to foods during processing. Anything fortified with a nutrient has extra amounts of that nutrient.

Sports Nutrition

What's the best food to eat before a competition?

What is creatine?

Do I need to eat more protein if I lift weights?

Do sports drinks, gels, and nutrition bars
really help my performance?

Does what I eat really affect my performance?

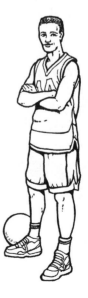

If you're reading this chapter, you probably participate in some type of sport or you plan to participate and want to improve your stamina or performance. First, let me congratulate you. If you've read Chapter 1 on the Dietary Guidelines, you know that you're already meeting a very important guideline—being physically active every day: "Get plenty of physical activity and reduce sedentary activities to promote health, psychological well-being, and a healthy body weight." Playing a sport and being physically active every day definitely does all of that and more. What you eat definitely can affect your ability

95

to perform, compete, and get the most out of your workout. As a teenager, you're still growing, so it's especially important to get all the nutrition that your body needs to grow and to fuel all of your activities.

EATING ENOUGH CALORIES

Fuel that machine. Your first priority is to eat enough calories so that you have enough energy to do the sports and activities that you love and keep growing (if you are still growing). Exercise uses a lot of calories, and you need to be sure that you feed your body so that it uses the calories efficiently. If you're not eating enough to support all of your activities, your body's metabolism (the rate at which you use calories) may slow down. That means you'll use fewer calories working out. Your body will choose to save its energy for more important things, such as making your heart beat and your lungs work.

HOW MANY CALORIES DO I NEED?

Using the table from Appendix A, Recommended Dietary Intakes, we could say that the average teen female needs about 2,000 calories/day and the average teen male needs about 2,300 calories/day. But remember, calorie needs are different for every person, depending on several individual factors. Your height, your weight, your age, your gender, and how much activity you do are all factors that affect how many calories you need each day.

There are some great websites with programs that let you enter your age, weight, activity level, and gender. Then the program tells you a recommended range of calories just for you. For example, the MyPyramid site is one that can do this.

Calories or energy needs include those required for basal metabolic rate (just enough to keep breathing), plus calories for the activities you do. As an athlete, you need to make sure you add enough calories to support your activity level. The amount you need depends on the type of activity you are doing.

Take a look at Appendix B to see how many calories you burn each hour doing various activities. Find the activities that you do and see how many calories each activity uses. Are you eating enough to support your sport?

For example, let's say you need about 2,000 calories each day to maintain your weight. If you are on the track team and run the equivalent of 1 hour each day, you need to add a factor for that activity. Let's suppose you weigh 155 pounds. At that weight, you could use up to 811 calories per hour running at the rate of 9 minutes/mile. You should then add those 811 calories to your daily requirement of 2,000. So you need to eat 2,811 calories per day to support that level of exercise.

> My daily calorie needs (from Appendix A) = A
> My activity calorie needs (from Appendix B) = B
> Total daily calorie needs = A + B

Remember, if you don't get enough calories, the long-term effects might be undesirable weight loss and, ultimately, reduced metabolism. A slower metabolism could have a negative effect on your performance and your overall health.

If you're trying to gain or lose weight, see Chapter 5 on weight management to find the best way to do this without affecting your performance.

Where Should My Calories Come From?

As mentioned in Chapter 2, calories come from three dietary sources: carbohydrates, protein, and fat. For the most part, the diets of physically active people need be no different from those of the general public. The recommendations are based on the Dietary Guidelines. That is, get about for 55–60 percent of total calories from carbohydrate (with about half of your carbohydrates coming from whole grains, fruits, and veggies), 20–35 percent or less from fat (especially healthy fats), and 15–20 percent from protein. Let's look at each of these separately.

CARBOHYDRATES

Carbohydrate is the main source of energy for your working muscles. You store carbohydrate in your muscles. When you exercise, your muscles use that stored carbohydrate, also known as glycogen, to do the work. That's why it is so important to include plenty of carbohydrate-containing foods in your diet. Dietary sources of carbohydrate include items from the blue strip of the food guide pyramid, such as breads, grains, pasta, fruits, fruit juices, and vegetables. In addition to energy, these foods supply lots of vitamins, minerals, and fiber. Remember that half of your grains should be whole grains.

What Is Carbohydrate Loading?

In the past, athletes were encouraged to follow a special "carbohydrate-loading" regimen the week before their competition. This process involved eating a low-carbohydrate diet for several days while training and then eating a high-carbohydrate diet for several days before the event. The theory behind carbohydrate loading is to load the muscles with glycogen (stored energy) so that when you are ready to exercise, there is plenty of glycogen available to get you through the event. See Table 8.1 for a sample carbohydrate loading regimen.

Table 8.1　Sample Carbohydrate-Loading Routine

- In the week before the competition, eat a normal diet (50–55 percent carbohydrate) for several days while training at your regular pace.

- Then for 2 days, gradually increase the carbohydrate to 65–70 percent of calories while reducing your training time.

- On the last day, rest while maintaining a high-carbohydrate diet.

- This modified regimen results in a large amount of glycogen stored in your muscles. It is important to rest your muscles the day before the event.

However, recent research has found that eating a low-carbohydrate diet for several days causes problems, such as hypoglycemia, nausea, dizziness, fatigue, and irritability. The research also shows the same glycogen-loading response with an easier and healthier regimen.

The process of carbohydrate loading is effective only for events of long duration, those lasting *longer than 90 minutes*. For short-term events, the process is not effective and may actually have some negative side effects. Carbohydrate needs water to be stored; in fact, for every gram of glycogen or carbohydrate that gets stored in the muscle, 3 grams of water also must be stored. This results in temporary "water weight" gain, which may make you feel bloated. For endurance athletes, this is okay because they sweat it out in the competition. For short-distance athletes, the extra weight may not be comfortable. Choose what is best for you based on the sport you play and how long you play it.

PROTEIN

Many athletes think they need to eat more protein in order to build muscle. The way to build muscle is to *exercise* the muscle. In fact, you simply can't get bigger muscles from eating any special diet. Muscles get bigger when they are worked. Aerobic exercise combined with strength training is the best way to do this. The energy needed for the work your muscle does is mostly supplied by carbohydrate, not protein. In fact, the average U.S. diet provides more than adequate amounts of protein. Most athletes need about 0.8 gram of protein per kilogram of body weight. Let's do the math and see what you need.

X = your weight in pounds
Y = your weight in kilograms (X divided by 2.2)
Y × 0.8 = grams of protein you need each day

Example: Someone weighing 155 pounds weighs about 70 kilograms (1 kilogram = 2.2 pounds). He or she needs 70 × 0.8 grams per kilogram = 56 grams of protein each day. This athlete could easily meet the 56 grams by consuming the following foods in one day.

Food Item	Protein (grams)
1 cup whole grain cereal with ½ cup low-fat milk	10 grams
1 ham and cheese sandwich	16 grams
3 ounces baked chicken	27 grams
½ cup brown rice	2 grams
1 glass low-fat milk	8 grams
2 tablespoons peanut butter with crackers	12 grams
Total	**75 grams**

You can see how easy it is to meet the recommendation for protein.

Shouldn't Athletes Eat More Protein Than Nonathletes?

Athletes who participate in endurance sports such as marathon biking or running may benefit from additional protein—perhaps 1–1.5 grams per kilogram of body weight. However, using our example, the requirement is still only 70–105 grams/day, which can be easily met with the typical U.S. diet.

Excess protein in the diet is stored as fat. The process of breaking down that extra protein produces nitrogen. Your kidneys have to get rid of, or excrete, any extra nitrogen in your diet. Therefore, a diet that is too high in protein can put a strain on your kidneys. In addition, a diet that is too high in protein can also cause calcium to be excreted by your body. You certainly don't want to be losing calcium, especially when calcium needs are so high during the teenage years. You could do some harm to your bones.

FAT

We need a certain amount of fat in our diets to provide some nutrients, to help us feel full, and to provide flavor to food. Athletes do not need any more or less fat in their diets than the general public. You probably wouldn't want to consume a meal or snack that is high in fat before an event or practice, because fat stays in the stomach longer than either carbohydrate or protein and can leave you feeling too full. See Chapter 2, "Find Your Fuel," for more information on fat.

WATER

Probably even more important than getting the right food in an athlete is making sure that athletes are well hydrated. A good eating plan for every athlete must include adequate fluids. The body requires water to cool itself, especially during periods of physical activity. When you exercise, your body cools itself by sweating. You can lose up to 6 cups of water in just 1 hour of continuous activity. Inadequate fluid intake can lead to dehydration and a decrease in performance. Besides decreasing your endurance, dehydration can cause serious effects such as heatstroke. Even a small amount of dehydration (1 percent of body weight or 1.5 pounds on a 150-pound person) can increase your risk of impaired performance and heat injury.

Warning Signs of Dehydration

Know the early signs of dehydration:

- Thirst
- Flushed skin
- Premature fatigue
- Increased body temperature
- Faster breathing and pulse rate
- Increased perception of effort
- Decreased exercise capacity

Later signs include the following:

- Dizziness
- Increased weakness
- Labored breathing with exercise

Fluid Replacement

Replace fluids during exercise to promote adequate hydration. Drink water rather than pouring it over your head. Drinking is the only way to rehydrate and cool your body from the inside out. Sports drinks are more appropriate than water for athletes engaged in moderate- to high-intensity exercise that lasts an hour or longer. Rehydrate after exercise by drinking enough fluid to replace fluid losses during exercise.*

How Much Water Do I Need?

Most people need about 6–8 glasses of water each day. Athletes should drink additional amounts before, during, and after exercise. Thirst is not the best indicator of hydration. Often, an athlete can be dehydrated and yet not feel thirsty. See Table 8.1 for tips on staying hydrated for exercise.

Table 8.1   Tips for Staying Hydrated*

- Begin exercise well-hydrated by drinking fluids during the day and within the hour before the exercise session.

- Replace sweat losses by drinking fluids regularly during exercise.

- Rehydrate after exercise to replace weight lost as fluid during exercise.

- Follow a personalized fluid replacement plan to prevent the consequences of excessive (more than 2 percent of body weight loss) dehydration, such as early fatigue, cardiovascular stress, increased risk of heat illness, and decreased performance.

---

*From Nutrition Facts handout "Exercise Hydration," Sports and Cardiovascular Nutritionists for the American Dietetic Association, April 2009.

---

* From the American Dietetic Association, "Hydrate Right," 2010.

If you ignore your thirst, you may start to show signs of mild dehydration. Your mouth may feel dry, and you may make less urine when you go to the bathroom. You may even feel dizzy or light-headed. These are sure signs that you need to start hydrating quickly. Mild dehydration is easy to correct. Start drinking those fluids. Severe dehydration can cause permanent damage to body systems. Don't let it get severe.

What about Sports Drinks?

Water is the best source of fluids for most athletes. It is readily absorbed and quickly replaces any lost fluids. For athletes exercising continuously for more than 60 minutes, a fluid with some extra nutrients may be a good idea. As you exercise, you lose water through your sweat. You also lose some minerals known as *electrolytes*. These minerals are important in fluid balance. They include sodium, potassium, and chloride. Athletes exercising more than 60 minutes or in extreme heat may need to replace fluid losses as well as electrolyte losses.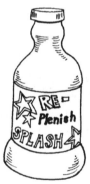

Diluted fruit juices, fruit drinks, and sports drinks can effectively replace lost fluid, including the electrolytes, as well as provide necessary energy to working muscles. Sports drinks usually have added potassium and sodium, the two common electrolytes lost in sweat. So, if you're working hard and really sweating, sports drinks may be a good idea. Full-strength juices should be avoided during exercise because they may cause cramping or nausea.

Sports drinks do have quite a few calories because of their relatively high sugar content. For recreational exercisers and those exercising less than 1 hour, the additional calories may not be necessary. Water is a better and more refreshing choice.

WHAT SHOULD YOU EAT *BEFORE* YOU EXERCISE?

When planning a meal before an event, there are several factors to consider:

- Choose foods that are familiar and comfortable for you. There's something to be said for the psychological effect of food. Right before your big game is not the time to try a new food.
- Choose high-carbohydrate, low-fat foods. Good choices include yogurt, bananas, apples, and oatmeal. These foods allow a steady stream of sugar in the blood and a steady source of energy for you.
- Avoid anything too sweet, such as soda and candy, which in some people causes a drop in blood sugar shortly after consumption. This low blood sugar, also known as hypoglycemia, can make you feel dizzy and nauseated.
- If you have 3–4 hours before your event, you can consume a relatively large meal.
- If you have less than 1 hour before your event, consume a small snack.
- If your competition is in the morning, you should still eat something. Don't skip breakfast. Your muscle glycogen stores are low after an overnight fast. A meal high in carbohydrate helps prevent low blood sugar.

WHAT CAN YOU EAT *DURING* EXERCISE?

If you are exercising for less than 60 minutes, you probably don't need to worry about eating while you're exercising. Just remember to stay hydrated. If your workout is lasting more than an hour, you may need more than just water to keep your muscles from getting too tired. Here are a few tips:*

---

* From the *Nutrition Fact Sheet, Sports and Cardiovascular Nutritionists for the American Dietetic Association*, April 2009.

- Drink sports drinks that contain carbohydrate and electrolytes, while avoiding ingredients that may slow digestion (such as fat and fiber).
- Choose easily digested, carbohydrate-rich foods during endurance events, for example, banana, bread or roll with jam or honey, sports foods (gels, gummy chews), or bite-sized pieces of low-fat granola or sports bars.
- Drink fluids consumed with carbohydrate gels or carbohydrate-rich foods to speed fuel transport to muscles.

WHAT SHOULD YOU EAT *AFTER* EXERCISE?

What you eat after your workout is important, too. You need to eat to refuel your body as well as to recover your muscles. That means you need calories (fuel), protein (for your muscles), and hydration with electrolytes (to replace lost fluid, sodium, and potassium). Here are a few tips from the *Nutrition Fact Sheet, Eating for Recovery, Sports and Cardiovascular Nutritionists with the American Dietetic Association*:

- Restore fluid and electrolytes (sodium and potassium) lost in sweat; weigh before and after exercise, and replenish what was lost.
- Replace muscle fuel (carbohydrate) utilized during practice.
- Provide protein to aid in repair of damaged muscle tissue and to stimulate development of new tissue.
- Begin nutrition recovery with a snack or meal within 15–60 minutes following practice or competition.

One of the simplest and cheapest foods to eat after your workout is a glass of chocolate milk. Milk is a fluid, so it hydrates you. Milk has protein, so it helps your muscles recover. Milk has some naturally occurring sodium in it as well. The chocolate can add some extra sugar and tastes pretty good, too.

Other post-workout snack ideas include the following: a smoothie made with yogurt and frozen berries, sports drink (carbohydrate, electrolyte, fluid) and a sports bar (carbohydrate, protein), or graham crackers with peanut butter and low-fat chocolate milk and a banana.

There are post-workout products that you can buy as well. You can buy specially formulated sports bars and powders that are marketed as "recovery" foods. These are generally safe, but expensive. Consider the simple foods first. A bagel and a banana work great. Often, these foods plus water are what you see offered at the end of a marathon for the athletes. We've also included a recipe to make your own energy bar (see Chapter 12).

ERGOGENIC AIDS

Whew! Ergogenic is a big word that refers to the foods, supplements, or other products that are marketed to athletes to try to convince them that they need this product to be better at their sport. Let's talk about some of the common ergogenic aids and whether or not they work, are worth the cost, or, most important, whether they are safe for you to use. Some are allowable and might help your performance; others are allowable but likely won't help you too much (too good to be true), and still others are actually unsafe.

Allowable and Might Help

- Caffeine
- Creatine
- Sports drinks, bars, and gels

Caffeine is known for its role as a stimulant to the central nervous system. Some athletes perceive that caffeine helps them feel as if they aren't working as hard. Newer research shows that moderate amounts of caffeine do not cause dehydration or electrolyte imbalance. **However, caffeine is still a restricted substance by the National Collegiate Athletic Association**, where a positive doping test is a caffeine level of 15 grams per milliliter of urine.

There are now many high-energy drinks on the market. These products contain large amounts of caffeine and can be dangerous when used in excess or in combination with stimulants, alcohol, or other unregulated herbals. Caffeine has many side effects, including anxiety, jitteriness, rapid heartbeat, gastrointestinal distress, and insomnia. For people who are not used to caffeine, the effects could actually impair their performance instead of improve it. The bottom line is that when rapid hydration is necessary, athletes should rely on noncaffeinated and nonalcoholic beverages.

Isn't Creatine Supposed to Improve Performance?

Creatine is one of the most widely marketed legal dietary supplements available today. Creatine is a naturally produced amino acid that is needed by the body to promote muscle movement during short, intense exercise. It can be purchased over the counter (nonprescription), but it also occurs naturally in food. For example, a pound of steak has about 2 grams of creatine. Initial research shows that creatine can be effective in some people during some types of exercise, resulting in a 5–10 percent increase in strength in short-term intermittent activities, such as sprinting. You store creatine in your muscles. However, once the muscle has enough creatine, any extra must be excreted in the urine. This can cause dehydration, resulting in muscle cramps and nausea.

The body uses creatine only during the first 20 or 30 seconds of an activity, so it doesn't appear to offer any real benefits for endurance athletes. Creatine really only offers a slight benefit to those athletes using it in conjunction with sport-specific training and very hard work. The most accomplished athletes have reported little or no benefits. As with other supplements, if your body isn't deficient in creatine in the first place, it may not need or benefit from additional amounts.

Although widely debated, creatine is generally considered safe for most healthy adults. The effects of long-term use of creatine remain unknown, but studies to date do not show any adverse effects in healthy adults from creatine supplementation Anyone taking or planning to take this supplement should consult a registered dietitian, preferably one with a sports nutrition background.

Sports Nutrition Bars

Like sports drinks, sports bars are readily available and being marketed to athletes, young and old. The bars are usually a concentrated source of energy. That is, they pack a lot of nutrition into a small bar. Their biggest benefit is convenience. You can tuck them into your backpack, waist pack, bike pack, or whatever, for a quick, high-energy snack or energy booster. Usually, the bars are high in calories (200–250 calories per bar), low in fat (2–3 grams per bar), and high in carbohydrate (45 grams per bar). Many are marketed as a pre-competition meal that optimizes performance. There is nothing magical in them that you couldn't consume on your own.

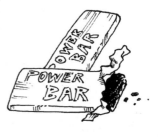

You can plan your own pre-competition meal with a similar composition. However, the convenience of these bars makes them an attractive option without harmful benefits. They are usually a better choice than a candy bar because they often have added vitamins, minerals, and protein that a candy bar does not have. A less expensive alternative is a breakfast bar or low-fat granola bar from your local supermarket.

Sports Gels

Another product marketed to athletes is sports gels or energy gels. These are individually packaged containers of carbohydrate gel that can be easily consumed before, during, or after an event. Basically, they are a fast-acting and easily digested carbohydrate (simple sugar). They are generally consumed during long training or events such as marathons. Eaten every 45 minutes or so, they can delay muscle fatigue, raise your blood sugar, and help your performance.

Sports gels come in many flavors. Some have added herbs and caffeine, so be sure to read the label carefully so you know what you are eating. Usually, athletes combine consumption of a gel with a lot of water to help digest it.

TOO GOOD TO BE TRUE

Like many weight-loss products, the majority of ergogenic aids currently on the market are in the "too good to be true" category, including amino acids, bee pollen, branched-chain amino acids, carnitine, chromium picolinate, cordyceps, coenzyme Q10, conjugated linoleic acid, cytochrome c, dihydroxyacetone, gamma oryzanol, ginseng, inosine, medium-chain triglycerides, pyruvate, oxygenated water, and vanadium.

To date, none of these products has been shown to enhance performance, and many have had adverse effects

What about Amino Acid Supplements and Protein Powders?

Protein is made up of different amino acids. If your diet is adequate in high-quality protein (from lean meat, fish, poultry, and milk), you are probably getting all the essential amino acids. If you are a vegetarian, you may need to pay closer attention to the sources of protein in your diet (see Chapter 7 on vegetarianism). Amino acids taken as supplements are beneficial only if the body is deficient in them in the first place. Amino acid supplements (such as ornithine and arginine) are marketed to athletes as necessary to build muscle. Remember that the way you truly build a muscle is to exercise that muscle.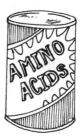

Amino acids taken in amounts that exceed your body's requirements are just excreted in the urine. There is no evidence that athletes need more of any amino acids than anyone else, nor is there compelling evidence that amino acid supplementation increases muscle mass or improves performance. Amino acid supplements can be a very expensive way to get your amino acids. Consider that a 4-ounce serving of chicken breast has 2,100 milligrams of **arginine** and costs less than a dollar. Most supplements provide just 85 milligrams of arginine in a serving and cost far more than that.

DON'T USE THESE PRODUCTS

The following is a list of dangerous products that are currently banned by the NCAA and other organizations. They are extremely dangerous and are not allowed in sports today: steroids—androstenedione, dehydroepiandrosterone, 19-norandrostenedione, 19-norandrostenediol, and other anabolic, androgenic steroids; *Tribulis terrestris*; ephedra; strychnine; and human growth hormone.

SUMMING UP SPORTS NUTRITION

Exercise is great for your emotional as well as physical well-being. A regular exercise program is the best way to help you feel better, sleep better, and look better. Make the most of your exercise program by eating a balanced diet. That means eating regularly (at least three meals a day plus snacks), planning your meals in advance, and choosing healthy meals and snacks at school, at home, and on the go. Try to resist the temptation to skip meals, snack on foods with little nutritional value, or experiment with fad diets and dietary supplements. The combination of eating right and exercising is a team that can't be beat! Go for it!

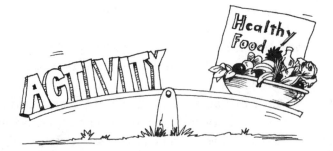

There's an app for this! Lots of cool apps for the athlete! You can download a training regimen for a 5k or even a marathon. You can track your training routine and progress with apps, too!

KEY TERMS AND DEFINITIONS

Metabolism: the rate at which your body burns calories

Basal metabolic rate: the amount of calories your body needs to maintain itself at rest

Glycogen: a storage form of carbohydrate

Hypoglycemia: low blood sugar, which can cause light-headedness, dizziness, and hunger

Endurance athlete: an athlete who trains or competes in events lasting longer than 60 minutes

Dehydration: a condition caused by inadequate fluid intake or excessive fluid loss that can cause dizziness or confusion

Electrolytes: minerals that are important in fluid balance in the body, including sodium and potassium

Ergogenic aids: foods, supplements, and other products that are marketed to athletes for their potential ability to enhance athletic performance

Funky Foods

Over 2,500 years ago, Hippocrates* said, "Let food be thy medicine and medicine be thy food."

So, is that what all the herbs and nutraceuticals, functional foods, bioengineered foods, and superfoods are about? It's tough to keep all of this straight. They sound like laboratory foods or fake food. Are they good for you? Should you put them in your body for fuel? The answer, unfortunately, is not simple.

Let's look at herbs, herbal remedies, and superfoods first and then take a look at functional foods that some are calling "nutraceuticals."

HERBAL REMEDIES

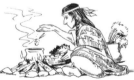

Herbs are plants that grow in the earth and are used to flavor food. They have been used historically as medicine. Herbal medicine is actually the oldest system of medicine known to humans. In early Indian cultures, a medicine man put together different mixtures of herbs and gave the mixture either to

---

* Hippocrates was a Greek physician born in 460 B.C. He is considered the "Father of Ancient Medicine." He believed that the body should be treated as a whole, not just as a series of parts.

ward off disease or to heal an ailment. Herbs are in the food chain and provide vitamins and minerals naturally.

It's interesting to see that herbal medicine today is considered to be an alternative medicine. So, what is alternative medicine? It's a practice of medicine that is not considered part of traditional medicine. It does not follow practices of traditional Western medicine and often uses herbs and specific foods instead of or with medicine. Just because you want to take herbs does not mean you cannot still go to your regular doctor. Many people just want to try to do something they think of as more "natural." Some people think that they might try herbs before getting a prescription drug from the doctor. A lot of us think that if something is natural, it must be healthier. This is not necessarily true.

Here are some different ways that people take herbs:

- Tea: either fresh or dried herbs can be used. You need to follow the directions on the package to make it properly.
- Powders and pills: the powder is pressed into pill form, or it is put into a capsule; a powder may be mixed with honey or into a food such as applesauce. Pills are convenient because the taste of medicinal herbs is usually bitter; you can take them with you and it's just like taking a vitamin.
- Tinctures: a tincture is a combination of alcohol and water that extracts the active ingredients of the herb into a liquid form. The use of alcohol helps preserve the herb's potency. Often the tincture is mixed with tea, or it may be made into a syrup by mixing it with a corn syrup or honey.
- Liniments and oils: these are for external use only, often for sore muscles, bruises, and skin problems.

Table 9.1 describes some of the more commonly purchased herbs today.

Table 9.1 Common Herbal Remedies and Their Uses			
	Scientific name	**Medicinal uses**	**More to know**
Echinacea	*Echinacea purpurea* (most commonly used)	Prevents and treats the common cold, flu, and infections. Helps strengthen the immune system. May be used for helping to heal skin wounds and acne.	Grows in North America in dry and open areas. May be used as tea, capsules, tablets, fluid extracts, and tinctures. FDA has not evaluated it for safety, effectiveness, or purity.
Ginkgo	*Ginkgo biloba*	Used for asthma, bronchitis, and fatigue. People take it hoping to improve brain function, but there is no proof of this.	Native to China but grown elsewhere today. Purchased as extract, capsules, or tinctures made from the leaves. Do not use if you have blood-clotting problems; do not take with aspirin. Do not take if pregnant or breastfeeding.
St. John's Wort	*Hypericum perforatum*	Used for depression, anxiety, and sleep problems. Used as an ointment for burns, wounds, and insect bites.	Native to Europe and now grown in the western part of the United States. Often taken as a pill or capsule. Tea can be made, and it is available as a tincture and extract. May interfere with medications taken for HIV. Do not take with

(continued on next page)

	Table 9.1 Common Herbal Remedies and Their Uses		
	Scientific name	Medicinal uses	More to know
St. John's Wort (cont'd)	*Hypericum perforatum*		antidepressants or sleeping medications. Birth control pills may not be as effective if taken with this. May cause increased sensitivity to sunlight.
Ginseng	*Panax quinquefolius*	Helps boost the immune system and improve overall health; lowers blood glucose and helps control symptoms of high blood pressure.	Grown in eastern and and central North America and China. When taken by mouth, usually considered safe. Some concern if taken for more than 3 months. Most common side effects are headache, sleep, and stomach problems.
Saw Palmetto	*Serenoa repens*	Often used for urinary problems resulting from an enlarged prostate gland. Also used for bladder problems, pelvic pain, decreased sex drive, hair loss, and hormone imbalance.	Native tree to southeastern United States. The dried berries are used and may be taken as pills, capsules, and extracts. May cause some mild stomach discomfort. Avoid if pregnant or breastfeeding; should not be given to small children.

(continued on next page)

	Scientific name	Medicinal uses	More to know
Table 9.1 Common Herbal Remedies and Their Uses			
Kava Kava	*Piper methysticum*	Usually used for anxiety, insomnia, and menopause.	Grown in the South Pacific. The root and underground stem can be made into beverages. It may be taken as a pill, capsule, or extract and used as a topical ointment. FDA warns that using this may cause severe liver damage. It may also interact with medications. DO NOT TAKE
Garlic	*Allium sativum*	Thought to help with heart disease by lowering cholesterol, decreasing atherosclerosis, and lowering blood pressure. Some feel this may prevent stomach and colon cancers.	Originally from Asia but is now grown throughout the world. Garlic may be eaten in its natural form but is also dehydrated and made into capsules, oils, and tincture. May cause bad breath, indigestion, and heartburn. May cause blood thinning; do not take 1 to 2 weeks before surgery. May interfere with a drug used to treat HIV.

(continued on next page)

Table 9.1 Common Herbal Remedies and Their Uses			
	Scientific name	Medicinal uses	More to know
Soy	Glycine max	Used to prevent or treat high cholesterol, menopause symptoms, hot flashes, memory problems, high blood pressure, breast and prostate cancers.	Soy is native to Asia and has been used in China for over 5,000 years. It is now grown throughout the world. The United States is a major producer. Soy is eaten today in many different forms, such as edamame, tofu, soy milk, and is used in many processed foods. It is frequently taken as a supplement as a tablet or capsule. Soy is considered safe for most people. May cause some minor stomach and bowel problems and, very rarely, breathing issues or rashes.

It's interesting that many of the medicines that pharmaceutical companies make come from herbal sources. For example, the laxative Senekot contains the herb senna. Many of us have taken Sudafed for allergies, but I bet you didn't know that it has the herb ephedra in it. The intent of herbal treatments is to try to make your body more efficient at healing itself naturally.

Herbal remedies are not considered to be the best choice by traditional doctors, health team members, and scientists in the United States. However, in many foreign countries, they are widely accepted and used.

So, what does this mean? Scientists in the United States are very cautious and careful. There are many regulatory agencies here, such as the Food and Drug Administration (FDA). The FDA monitors all new drugs before they are allowed to be sold in the United States. There is a lengthy scientific process that a scientist or drug company must go through before a drug can be sold to people. Part of this process is called "clinical trials," which means that doctors give the drugs to people in controlled studies.

Although many of the herbal remedies are considered safe, they have not gone through this same testing process. Scientists feel that they do not know exactly how these herbal remedies actually work or what kind of dosage (how much of the herb) should be given. Did you know that the potency of an herb actual depends on the crop itself? This means that when you buy one brand you may get one amount of the herb; if you buy another brand, you might get a different amount. Another problem according to scientists is that the FDA does not currently regulate herbs. There is no quality control. It's like going to the gas station and filling up the tanks, but you're not sure what gas you're actually getting or how much you're getting.

Paul Sanders, ND, PhD, a Professor at the Canadian College of Naturopathic Medicine states: "Natural is not synonymous with safe." In other words, just because something is called "natural," it isn't necessarily good for you. Some herbs have been found to be contaminated or even contain prescription drugs. You should think carefully before taking these. They may be harmful if taken for extended periods or in large quantities. Herbs work slowly, so you need to be very careful before increasing how much you take. The bottom line is this: make sure that you tell your doctor exactly what you are taking and how much. Check out Table 9.2 before taking herbal remedies

FUNCTIONAL FOODS

These are sometimes called nutraceutical or bioengineered foods. The one thing to remember is that they are foods—not vitamin or mineral supplements. There are many different definitions, but here's one from the Institute of Medicine, a branch of the National Acad-

---

Table 9.2   Facts to Consider before Using Herbal Remedies

Dos
Do find out exactly what you are taking.

- Do look for "USP" on the label. This stands for U.S. Pharmacopeia, which is an organization that checks for uniformity of products.
- Do tell your doctor what you are taking (there is a book that lists all the herbs and interactions or complications that may occur).
- Do buy herbs that are manufactured by reputable companies.
- Do read the small print for warnings.
- Do stop taking immediately if you have any side effects.

Don'ts
- Don't stop taking a prescription drug in order to try an herbal remedy in its place.
- Don't use herbs if you're pregnant or breastfeeding.
- Don't exceed recommended dosages.
- Don't use herbs to treat serious illnesses.

---

emy of Sciences: "Any modified food or food ingredient that may provide a health benefit beyond the traditional nutrients it contains."

This really means that almost all foods could be considered functional because, when you think about it, all foods have some health benefit, right? Table 9.3 describes some of the common food components and tells how they can benefit your health. The table contains a lot of information. But when you look at the food-component column, many everyday foods that we eat are listed. So, what's the deal with calling things functional foods?

Let's categorize functional foods to clear some things up:

Conventional or Natural Foods: Food in its original state (e.g., fruits, vegetables, meat, fish)

Modified Foods: Food to which something has been added or food that has been fortified with a nutrient added to make the food even more nutritious (e.g., orange juice with calcium)

Manufactured Foods: Food developed by food companies (sport drinks, sports bars)

	Table 9.3 Functional Foods and Their Health Benefits		
Food Component	**Food Ingredient**	**Health Source**	**Benefits**
Carotenoids	Carrots	Antioxidant	Promotes healthy cells and lessens risk of cancer and heart disease
Lutein (a carotenoid)	Green vegetables		May reduce the risk of macular degeneration (may promote healthy vision)
Lycopene	Tomatoes	Antioxidant	May reduce risk of prostate cancer
Calcium	Milk and dairy products		Improves bone health and decreases risk of osteoporosis
Dietary fiber (beta glucan)	Oats		Reduces risk of heart disease
Dietary fiber (insoluble fiber)	Wheat bran		May reduce risk of breast or colon cancer
Fatty acids (omega-3 fatty acids)	Salmon and other fatty fish		May reduce risk of heart disease and improve mental and visual functions
Fatty acids (conjugated linoleic acid, or CLA)	Cheese and meat		May improve body composition; may reduce risk of certain cancers
Flavonoids	Fruits and vegetables	Antioxidant	May reduce risk of heart disease and cancer

(continued on next page)

	Table 9.3 Functional Foods and Their Health Benefits		
Food Component	**Food Ingredient**	**Health Source**	**Benefits**
Glucosinolates, indoles, isothiocyanates	Broccoli, kale, cauliflower		May reduce risk cancer
Prebiotics and probiotics	Jerusalem artichokes, shallots, onion powder		May improve gastrointestinal health
Prebiotics and probiotics (lactobacillus)	Yogurt		May improve lactose intolerance and gastrointestinal health
Soy proteins (isoflavones)	Soybeans and soy foods		May reduce menopausal symptoms
Thiols (diallyl sulfide)	Garlic, onions, olives, leeks, scallions		Lowers LDL (low-density lipoproteins)
Tannins (proantho-cyanidins)	Cranberry products		May improve urinary tract health

CONVENTIONAL OR NATURAL FOODS

We'll talk about what we think of as natural foods first. Let's look at milk. Milk has calcium in it naturally, and we know that calcium is important for our bones and also in the fight against osteoporosis (bone degeneration). Oranges could also be considered a functional food. They are naturally a good source of vitamin C. We know that vitamin C is an antioxidant and that antioxidants are important in reducing the risk of cancer and heart disease. (See Chapter 3 to learn more about calcium and antioxidants.) So we just need to eat foods that are good for us, right? Not necessarily.

People today are talking about "superfoods." There are many books written about these foods. Let's take a look at some of the really popular superfoods. We like the list that WebMD's Nutrition Director, Kathleen Zelman, MPH, RD, LD, came up with, but we added some of our own. They can be found in Table 9.4.

FORTIFIED FOODS

As mentioned previously, fortified food is a food to which something has been added. Some food companies are now taking advantage of the consumer's interest in health and adding specific food components associated with health benefits. For example, calcium has been added to orange juice. You can buy Special K Plus cereal with additional calcium and iron. Check out in the grocery stores all the new drinks that have herbs in them. Food companies are fortifying items with these functional attributes or parts of food that are considered to be healthy. Actually, this makes sense when we go back to that definition of functional foods. The definition says that a food has been modified.

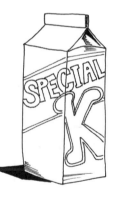

MANUFACTURED FOODS

Now let's take a look at manufactured foods. These are also of big interest to food companies. Sports nutrition really has brought bio-engineered foods into the forefront. What's an energy bar? It looks

Table 9.4 Superfoods		
Food	**Why it's good**	**Interesting facts**
– Super Dairy – Low-fat or fat-free plain yogurt *Recipe:* Blueberry parfait*	High in calcium, good source of protein and potassium. Often tolerated better by people who are lactose-intolerant.	Is a probiotic and produces lactic acid. Boosts the immune sytem and enhances intestinal health.
– Super Meats – Beans *Recipe:* David's Three-Alarm Chili*	Insoluble and soluble fiber. Also a good source of protein.	Good for your heart; helps reduce LDL cholesterol.
Eggs *Recipe:* Family Frittata*	Very nutritious, great source of protein, and packed with vitamins and minerals. Inexpensive.	Elizabeth Ward, MS, RD, author of *The Pocket Idiot's Guide to the New Food Pyramids*, states, "Studies show if you eat eggs at breakfast, you may eat fewer calories during the day and lose weight without significantly affecting cholesterol levels."
Nuts *Recipe:* Banana Bran Muffins*	Good source of protein, fiber, and heart-healthy fats. Contain antioxidants.	Need to watch portions so that you do not overeat. Make your own snack packs.

(continued on next page)

Table 9.4 Superfoods		
Food	**Why it's good**	**Interesting facts**
– Super Meats – *(cont'd)* Salmon *Recipe:* Salmon Cakes*	Rich in omega-3 fatty acids. Great source of protein.	A fatty fish, but good fat. Helps brain functioning as well as your heart. Some research indicates that it may help with weight loss.
Soy *Recipe:* Banana Shake*	Richest source of protein of any legume. Contains phytoestrogens and disease-fighting phytonutrients.	Soy nuts might be a good snack option. Ever tried edamame? Quite the interesting veggie!
– Super Fruits *and Veggies –* Acai	Lots of antioxidants and essential fatty acids.	Grown in Brazil; the berries deteriorate quickly. We usually purchase as juice.
Berries *Recipe:* Blueberry Parfait*	Great source of antioxidants, phytochemicals; high in fiber and low in sugar.	Blueberries are considered the star, but cranberries, blackberries, strawberries, and raspberries are all good.
Broccoli *Recipe:* Pasta with Chicken and Broccoli*	Great source of vitamins A (beta-carotene) and C.	Very filling and low in calories. Can eat raw or cooked.

(continued on next page)

Table 9.4 Superfoods		
Food	**Why it's good**	**Interesting facts**
– Super Fruits and Veggies – (cont'd)		
Kiwi *Recipe:* Fruit Concoction*	Extremely nutrient dense. Has the most vitamin C of any fruit; contains lutein.	Can also eat the skin; good source of fiber and nutrients.
Pomegranates	Rich in vitamin C and antioxidants.	Add some seeds to a salad, or try the juice.
Sweet potatoes *Recipe:* Sweet Potato Pudding*	Excellent source of vitamins A and C, calcium, potassium, and fiber.	Eat instead of white potatoes; they have lots more fiber.
– Super Grains –		
Barley *Recipe:* Barley and Mushroom Risotto*	Great source of insoluble and soluble fiber. Rich in B vitamins and antioxidants.	Slightly sweet taste; great to add to salads.
Oats *Recipe:* Colleen's Granola	Excellent source of soluble and insoluble fiber. Good source of vitamins B and E and minerals calcium, magnesium, and potassium.	Reduces cholesterol.

(continued on next page)

Table 9.4	Superfoods	
Food	**Why it's good**	**Interesting facts**
– Super Grains – *(cont'd)*		
Quinoa *Recipe:* Quinoa and Black Bean Salad*	An ancient whole grain; has more protein than any other grain. Great source of fiber and iron.	Easy to prepare. Why not try some other ancient grains that are increasing in popularity: amaranth, barley, millet, buckwheat, and flax?
* See Chapter 12.		

like a candy bar; some energy bars even taste like candy bars, but guess what? It isn't a candy bar. Food companies have put together different ingredients and bioengineered them into something that tastes good and yet has specific percentages of protein, fat, and carbo-hydrate—supposedly, to help athletes perform at their best. Food companies are aware that people are concerned about health and the impact of nutrition. As a result, they are making lots of different manufactured food items, and people are buying them up like crazy. There is spaghetti for athletes that is supposedly better because it has been bioengineered to be just right for maximum performance. Lots of food items are available for athletes to purchase.

THE BOTTOM LINE

Functional foods are big business for companies. Many people say that these functional foods are the "next generation of healthy prod-ucts." People want to improve their health, not change how they eat.

So how does this translate? You want to eat something that's tasty, makes you feel better, is better for you, and helps you perform better too. Wow! That's a lot for a food to do or "claim" to do.

So, when we talk about functional foods, the health "claim" is where it's at. There has to be a health claim on the label. For example, the health claim for oatmeal is this: "Sol-uble fiber from oatmeal as part of a low saturated fat, low cholesterol diet may reduce the risk of heart disease." These health claims have to be real and proven, but there are many questions about what gov-ernment agencies are regu-lating these new and emerg-ing food components or ingredients. See Chapter 11 for more information on health claims.

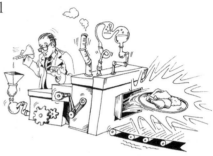

Now that food companies know that functional foods are benefi-cial for our health, they are adding some of these components to foods that are already popular (such as adding calcium to orange juice), or they are making up new foods. For example, food manufac-turers are even creating butter-like spreads from healthy oils. Ameri-cans like the taste of butter but would like a healthy option. Olive oil is a "good" fat. Why not try Olivio spread? If you don't quite like that taste, try Olivio Spreadable Butter. This is a combination of butter and olive and canola oils. Want another option? Try Smart Balance Omega Plus—that's a mouthful! This is a combination of oils and has omega-3 fatty acids. Have your "butter" and improve your blood lipids at the same time!

Yikes! There are so many choices out there. *Proceed with caution*: do not substitute any foods or functional foods for medication.

Should I buy these products? You need to take a look at your nutritional status. You also need to look at the cost of these products. They are usually expensive. If you're getting the recommended number of servings according to the food guide pyramid, you probably don't need to spend money on this extra nutrition.

So you, as the consumer, need to decide whether or not it is financially worth it for you to pay the additional cost. The U.S. Department of Agriculture and the FDA are working hard to keep up with the growing interest and manufacturing of these functional foods. This is new territory, so there are not all the safeguards built in as there are with our traditional food supply. Getting back to the idea of our bodies being like cars, we could find recalls of some of these products!

KEY TERMS AND DEFINITIONS

Remedies: treatments for diseases or illnesses

Food chain: a system for food that grows and eventually reaches the consumer. Food may go through many steps before reaching the consumer, such as processing, manufacturing, and distribution

Traditional medicine: In Western medicine, a patient is seen by a physician and diagnosed and treated by what Americans believe to be normal means, that is, antibiotics, surgery, and recognized medications. Traditional medicine is often compared to Eastern or Chinese medicine, whereby alternative approaches, such as herbal remedies and acupuncture, are used.

Quality control: a check-and-balance system that is put in place to ensure that the quality and consistency of a product or service are met and maintained

Osteoporosis: a condition in which bones are weak and break easily

Antioxidants: substances that have been shown to help the body cells fight diseases such as cancer and heart disease

Phytonutrients: nutrients or chemicals that come from plants and are thought to promote health. They are not essential for life and are often referred to as phytochemicals.

Fast Facts on Fast Foods

Gotta have fries? Big Mac attack? Whether it's the stop after the game, where you go to meet up with your friends, or a quick meal stop in between activities, fast food is a part of American lives. And although it's not always the healthiest choice, it is unrealistic to say that you'll never eat in a fast-food restaurant again. Rather, fast food, like any food, can be part of a healthy lifestyle. It just takes a little know-how and willingness on your part to make a few changes.

WHY IS FAST FOOD CONSIDERED UNHEALTHY?

Although not all fast food is unhealthy, most fast-food choices tend to be high in fat, sodium, sugar, and calories. At the same time, fast-food choices are usually low in fiber and low in vitamins A and C, primarily as a result of the lack of fruit and vegetable choices on the menu.

Can you have your fries and eat them, too? Absolutely. But you need to balance your choices so that the end result is a diet still in keeping with the Dietary Guidelines (see Chapter 1.). If you eat at fast-food restaurants only occasionally (i.e., once or twice a month), it's probably not quite so important to make healthier selections while you're there. However, if you're there often enough that they know your order; you probably need to read this chapter. Fast food is likely a significant contributor of fat, sodium, and calories to your diet. It also could be taking the place of more nutritious foods in your diet.

WHAT TO WATCH OUT FOR WHEN EATING OUT

Here are some things to keep in mind when eating out.

1. *Watch out for "mega-sizing."*
    Super size, mega size, Humongo Gulp. Why do people seem to want such big servings these days? Usually, these restaurants entice you with the package deal, so that, for just a little more money, you get a lot more food—whether you need it or not. Be discriminating. Are you really that hungry? Why not share your mega meal with your buddy and really save some money? Or just get the smaller versions of these items. You'll end up spending less money, and you'll still feel satisfied.

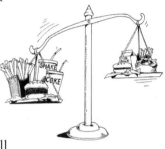

2. *Chicken and fish are not always the best choices.*
    We tend to think poultry and fish are better for us than red meat. It's not necessarily so, as Table 10.1 shows. Fast-food restaurants often bread and fry chicken and fish. The end product can have as much or more fat and calories than a hamburger. Choose chicken or fish that is broiled, baked, or grilled. If you're not sure how it's prepared, ask. Most fast-food restaurants have the nutrient content of their menu items either right in the restaurant or certainly on their website. There are even apps for your cell phone that can tell you the nutrient info for some fast-food chains.

3. *Order a side salad once in a while instead of fries.*
    Many restaurants offer salads on the menu now. It's a great way to "beef" up your vegetable intake without the beef. Watch out, though. Salads can be a big calorie buster too. Heavy dressings

Table 10.1 How a Hamburger Compares to Other Fast-Food Choices		
Fast-Food Item	**Grams of Fat**	**Calories per Serving**
Burger King Chicken Sandwich	36	685
McDonalds Filet-O-Fish	24	370
KFC Colonel's Chicken Sandwich	24	482
Taco Bell Chicken Burrito	12	334
McDonald's Regular Hamburger	8	255

and added items in salads, such as crispy strips, croutons, nuts, etc., can make a salad have as many calories as a burger and fries—or even more. Just two ounces of ranch dressing (about one of those packets) provides 20 grams of fat. That's as much as in a quarter-pounder. Go for the "lite" or reduced-fat dressings, or use less of the heavier ones. Make sure that your salad is heavier on the veggies than on the extras.

4. *Specialty coffees.*
   Coffee shops can be a fun place to hang out and have a cup of joe with your buddies. Although a cup of coffee and a muffin as a snack sounds pretty good, the choices available these days can turn a cup of coffee and a muffin into a whole meal in terms of calories—but perhaps not a whole meal in terms of nutrition.

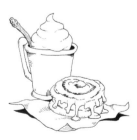

To increase your intake of other food groups, try ordering some 100 percent fruit juice or fat-free milk with your meal. You could also have an egg on your bagel instead of cream cheese, to get a little protein. As for the coffee, be sure that you know what you are getting when you place your order. Although coffee and tea alone don't have any calories, they do have caffeine. Caffeine can act as a diuretic, making you lose water from your body. In addition, caffeine can increase your heart rate and cause stomach upset, nausea, and headaches. Finally, once you start adding things to your coffee, such as milk and sugar, you can end up with some unwanted calories or fat.

2 teaspoons sugar	+30 calories
2 tablespoons whole milk	+20 calories
2 tablespoons cream	+40 calories

Specialty or gourmet coffees such as lattes can also pack a calorie and fat punch as a result of added sugars and fat in the whole milk or cream. However, if ordered with fat-free (skim) milk, these drinks can actually provide a fair amount of protein and calcium.

5. *Try different menu items.*
   Many fast-food restaurants offer more than just burgers and fries. There are often nutritious choices, such as soup, baked potatoes, salads, yogurt, milk, or bagels.

6. *Choose a nutritious thirst quencher.*
   Teens today are getting over 10 percent of their daily calories from soda and other sweetened beverages.* The soft drink industry is a huge one, spending billions of advertising dollars to get you to choose their product. Regardless of the flavor or the man-

---

* The percentage of calories from sweetened beverages for youth aged 2–18 years has increased steadily: from 4.8 percent of total calories (1977–1978) to 6.1 percent (1989–1991) to 8.5 percent (1994–1996) to 10.3 percent of daily calories in 1999–2001. Nielsen S. J. and Popkin, B. M. Changes in Beverage Intake between 1977 and 2001. *Am. J. Prev. Med.* 2004;27(3):205–210.

ufacturer of the product, most soft drinks
are nutritionally about the same. They
provide lots of calories in the form of
added sugar, but few other nutrients.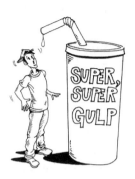
Some sodas, especially cola bever-
ages, also contain caffeine, an addictive stimulant that you don't need.
Finally, many soft drinks (including
diet soft drinks) contain quite a bit of
the mineral phosphorus. Excess amounts
of the form of phosphorus found in colas
and root beer may cause your body to lose calcium. We discussed the importance of calcium in Chapter 3 and
how it helps keep your bones strong.

Here are a few tips on choosing your thirst quencher. Know what
you are getting and think about other choices.

Soda: If you are going to drink soda, know that most 12-ounce
cans (except diet soft drinks) have about 150 calories or so, all
from added sugar. There may be caffeine, too. Read the label.

Water: Water is the best thirst quencher. It hydrates your body
quickly. Bottled, spring, or right from the tap, it's great stuff.

Sports drinks: Sports drinks, such as Gatorade, are a little better
than soda. They usually have some added sodium and potassium
to replenish those minerals lost during exercise. Still, all of the
calories come from added sugar. If you're not working out and not
sweating a lot, you do just as well with water.

Juice: For the same amount of calories as soda, you could have
100 percent fruit juice and get some vitamins in your diet. These
drinks usually have vitamin C, and now some juices have added
calcium.

Milk: Again, for similar calories as a soda, you can have milk and
get calcium, vitamin D, and complete protein. It's not a bad deal.

Iced-coffee smoothie drinks made with whole milk: Depending on how you order it, an iced-coffee smoothie can have 230 calories (a 16-ounce drink made with fat-free milk and sugar) to 410 calories (a 16-ounce drink made with cream and sugar).

Fruit smoothies made with fruit, sugar, and ice: If made with real fruit (ask if you're not sure), these drinks are a refreshing way to punch up your fruit intake. But for those of you watching your calories, know that these can have plenty, especially if sugar is added. Check out Table 10.2 to compare your favorite beverages.

HOW TO MAKE BETTER FAST-FOOD CHOICES

Take a look at Table 10.3 and try to take some of the suggestions into consideration when you visit your favorite fast-food restaurant. Remember that all foods can fit into your meal plan. It's just a matter of how often you choose certain foods and what else you eat along with them that make the difference. You can see that by just changing the side item or the beverage, you can save lots of calories and gain lots of nutritional value.

In Chapter 11, we emphasize meal planning and thinking about your day. This is good advice when you know you'll be eating out later. If you know you're going to be eating dinner at a fast-food restaurant, try to eat more foods during the day that are high in vitamins and fiber. Have some extra fruit, veggies, and whole grains for breakfast and lunch, keeping your fat intake a little lower, when you know you'll be at a fast-food restaurant later.

Sometimes, though, you just can't plan ahead. The day got away, practice got out late, and Mom didn't have time to get something on the table. So you end up going out for dinner. This is fairly common practice in busy households these days. Just adjust your intake the next day, again emphasizing the fruits, vegetables, and whole grains. Balance is the key to good nutrition and health.

Table 10.2 The Big Beverage Comparison				
Beverage (16-Ounce Serving)	Calories	Added Sugar in Grams	Fat in Grams	Other Nutrients
Cola soft drink	186	47	0	None
Sports drink (Gatorade)	113	29	0	Potassium, sodium
Iced-coffee smoothie made with whole milk	260	51	4	Calcium 15% (% Daily Value)* Vitamin A 2% (% Daily Value)*
Fruit smoothie	280	63	0	Vitamin C 45% (% Daily Value)* 1 gram fiber
Low-fat milk	190	0	5	Calcium 558 milligrams, 15 grams protein; also contains potassium, sodium, vitamin A
Orange juice	204	0	0	Vitamin C, potassium, folic acid

* Daily value (on a food label) refers to how the food contributes to your overall daily intake; see Chapter 12 for more information on food labels.

Table 10.3 Better Fast-Food Choices		
Instead of this	**Try this**	**Why?**
For Lunch or Dinner		
At McDonald's		
Double cheeseburger, large fries, and a large coke	Regular cheeseburger, small fries, side salad, and low-fat milk	You'll save 790 calories, and you'll be adding more calcium, more fiber, and vitamins.
At Taco Bell		
Nacho grande with sour cream and a large soda	2 crisp tacos with lettuce and tomato and a bottle of water	You'll save 740 calories and reduce your meal in fat and saturated fat.
At Wendy's		
BBQ Bacon crispy deluxe sandwich with fries and a Frosty	BBQ Bacon crispy deluxe sandwich with side salad and a chocolate milk	You'll save 529 calories, less saturated fat, more fiber and vitamins.
At KFC		
Extra crispy chicken breast with potato wedges and a 16-ounce soda	Original recipe chicken breast with mashed potatoes (no gravy) and low-fat milk	You'll save 390 calories and lots of fat, and you'll add calcium to your meal.
At Subway Footlong chicken bacon ranch with chips and a soda	6-inch sweet onion chicken teriyaki with baked chips and a low-fat milk	You'll save 865 calories, and you'll add more calcium and vitamin D to your meal.
For Breakfast		
At McDonalds		
Sausage McGriddle and a medium orange juice	Egg McMuffin and a medium orange juice	You'll save 290 calories and reduce the saturated fat in your meal.

Table 10.3 Better Fast-Food Choices		
Instead of this	**Try this**	**Why?**
For Breakfast		
At Burger King		
Breakfast sausage biscuit sandwich and orange juice	Egg and cheese Croissanwich and orange juice	You will save 260 calories and lots of fat.
At Starbucks		
20-ounce cinnamon dolce latte made with 2-percent milk and a cinnamon chip scone	Cinnamon dolce latte (16-ounce with nonfat milk) and Starbucks perfect oatmeal with brown sugar	You will save 420 calories and add fiber and whole grain to your meal.
At Chick-fil-A		
A chicken breakfast burrito with hash browns	Chicken minis with a yogurt parfait	You will save 240 calories and add protein, calcium, and vitamin C to your meal.

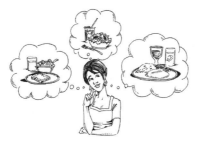

APP There's an app for this. You can download apps that tell you the nutrition information on all of your favorite fast-food menu items. This can really help you make an educated decision the next time you visit the restaurant.

KEY TERMS AND DEFINITIONS

Caffeine: an addictive stimulant found in coffees, teas, cola beverages, and chocolate. Can cause the body to lose fluids and cause side effects such as headache, stomach upset, and nausea

Diuretic: substance that increases urination and promotes water to be lost from the body

Phosphorus: a mineral that is involved in maintenance of bone

Smoothie: a blenderized drink

Meal Planning

There are a lot of things we've been talking about to keep your body, this fine-tuned machine, running as efficiently as possible. Something you want to remember is that you don't want to run out of gas. It seems pretty obvious—your body needs fuel to run.

We've discussed the food guide pyramid. The pyramid tells you the types and amounts of food that you should have throughout the day. But how do you do that? Usually, we think that three meals a day is normal, but what's normal for one person may not be right for someone else. Some people prefer to eat several small meals throughout the day. You may even know 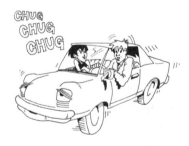 people who eat just one large meal a day. But we are talking about *good* nutrition. It's best to fuel your body throughout the day—you really do want to have at least three meals a day.

BREAKFAST

Breakfast is probably the most important meal of the day. You had dinner and maybe a bedtime snack, but then you were sleeping for, hopefully, 8 to 12 hours. Your body needs fuel to get started the next morning. Research studies prove that kids do better on tests, are more attentive and alert, are more motivated, are able to concentrate better, and have more energy when they've eaten breakfast. The Dietary Guidelines Advisory Committee for 2010 found that "Moderate evidence suggests that children who do not eat breakfast are at increased risk of overweight and obesity. The evidence is stronger for adolescents." So chances are, if you eat breakfast, you are less likely to be overweight or obese. That's a lot for a meal to do. But it does.

What should you have for breakfast? You need to get about 25–33 percent of your daily calories from breakfast. There are certain foods that you think of as breakfast foods, but guess what? There is no magic to these foods.

Traditional Breakfast Foods

Eggs • Waffles • Cereal • Pancakes • Bacon • Toast • Yogurt •
Toaster tarts• Sausage • Biscuits and gravy • Donuts • Fruit •
Juice • Bagel

Of course, you don't want to forget the food guide pyramid. It would be great to get some foods from the different categories. Let's put together some healthy choices. A traditional breakfast might consist of eggs, toast, juice, and milk. Table 11.1 shows the breakdown. If you're in a hurry, you might try the option in Table 11.2: an apple, a bagel, and a yogurt.

HOW DOES THIS STACK UP?

We are using 2,000 calories/day for an average teen female and 2,300 calories/day for an average teen male. But remember, calorie needs are different for every person depending on several individual factors. Your height, your weight, your age, your gender, and how much activity you do are all factors that affect how many calories you need each day.

Table 11.1 A Traditional Breakfast			
Food Item	Pyramid	Calories	What's good about It?
1 cup orange juice	1 serving fruit	112	Great source of vitamin C
2 scrambled eggs	1 serving meat, poultry, etc.	199	Excellent protein source
2 slices whole-wheat toast with margarine	2 servings bread, cereals, etc. 1 serving fats, oils, sweets	198	Source of dietary fiber, B vitamins, and iron
1 cup low-fat milk	1 serving milk, yogurt, cheese	103	Great source of calcium
Total calories		612	

How does this stack up?	Percentage of Calories Required for the day
Teen female	31%
Teen male	27%

Now, maybe you're not a big breakfast eater, or maybe you like something a little different. What about pizza or a sandwich? See Table 11.3 for some good options.

There really are a lot of different options for breakfast. Also, many schools have breakfast programs. So why not take advantage? If you have a free first or second period, grab a friend and get something to eat.

LUNCH

Now that we have breakfast taken care of, let's check out lunch. Depending on when you had breakfast, you're probably starting to get

Table 11.2 A Breakfast Option for Someone in a Hurry			
Food Item	**Pyramid**	**Calories**	**What's Good about It?**
1 Odwala Chocolate Chip Peanut Butter Bar	2 servings grains	219	Good source of fiber and protein
12 ounces of orange juice	2 servings fruit	180	Great source of vitamin C
1 large banana	1½ servings fruit	109	Good source of fiber
1 piece string cheese	1 ounce of meat or beans	80	Good source of protein and 150 milligrams of calcium
Total Calories		**588**	

How does this stack up?	Percentage of Calories Required for the day
Teen female	29%
Teen male	26%

hungry around 11 or so. Hear any of that growling in your stomach? Those noises are telling you that you need to put something in your stomach to keep you going.

It doesn't matter if you bag lunch or buy it or eat it at home. Just do it. You should get about 33 percent of your daily calories from lunch. Don't forget the food groups on the food guide pyramid. Lunch is an easy time for you to get foods from most of the different groups. Don't skimp. You are growing and active, so you need to get that fuel. Without a good lunch, you may find yourself dragging and unable to pay attention by the time your last class rolls around.

Table 11.3 Something a Little Different for Breakfast			
Food Item	**Pyramid**	**Calories**	**What's Good about It?**
2 slices of pizza	2 servings bread, cereal, etc.; 1 serving vegetables; 8 servings milk, yogurt, cheese	576	Tastes great. You are getting servings from three food groups. You have 29% of your calories if you're a and 25% if you're a male.
Ham and cheese sandwich	2 servings bread, cereal, etc.; 1 serving meat, poultry, etc.; ½ serving milk, yogurt, cheese; ½ serving fats, oils, sweets	399	Can take and eat on your way. You're getting foods from three good groups. You have 19% of your calories if you're a female and 16% if you're a male. Add a cup of 1% milk and a cup of orange juice, and you have a complete breakfast.
Beef and bean burrito	1 serving bread, cereal, etc.; ½ serving meat, poultry, etc.; ½ serving fats, oils, sweets	254	Good source of fiber. For the road. You have 12% of your calories if you're a female and 10% if you're a male.

At School

Most schools participate in the USDA-funded National School Lunch Program. If you buy your lunch at school and you choose the complete meal option, you're getting a well-balanced meal and an economical option. Table 11.4 gives an example from the National School Lunch Program.

Table 11.4. Example of a Typical School Lunch	
Food Item	**Pyramid**
Teriyaki chicken sandwich on a whole-grain bun with lettuce and tomato	Bread, cereal, etc.; meat, poultry, etc.; vegetable
French fries	Vegetable
Choice of fruit	Fruit
Chocolate milk	Milk, yogurt, cheese

The National School Lunch Program must also meet the U.S. Dietary Guidelines for Americans, so your meal has 30 percent or less of the calories from fat and 10 percent or less from saturated fat. Yes, this really is true. Often, foods are specially developed so that they meet these requirements: so your chicken nuggets at school lunch most likely do not have the same nutritional profile as what you get at a fast-food chain. The National School Lunch Program is also required to give 33 percent of the calories you need for the day. If you choose this option, you've made a good choice.

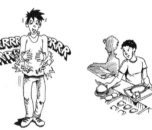

Most of the secondary schools offer à la carte items in addition to the complete meal plan. You can choose whatever you want. Sometimes it's easy to get off track and just buy fries, cookies, and juice. This may taste good, but you're getting only vegetables and fruit from the pyramid. Try to make some better choices. Why not grab a "submarine" sandwich, cookies, and juice? You're still getting the vegetables (lettuce and tomato on the sub) and fruit, but you also have bread, cereal, grains, and meat. It's important to have some protein; it sticks with you for a longer time. Your stomach won't be growling before school gets out.

Bag It.

It's easy to pack a healthy lunch that is also satisfying. You might be a traditionalist and like the usual—a sandwich, chips, fruit—and you can purchase milk. Check Table 11.5 to see how this lunch stacks up.

If you're not so traditional and like some funky foods, see Table 11.6 for some good suggestions that also add variety and convenience.

Table 11.5 A Traditional Lunch			
Food Item	**Pyramid**	**Calories**	**What's Good about It?**
Turkey sandwich on whole-wheat bread with lettuce and tomato, pretzels, low-fat granola bar, banana, nonfat milk	4 servings bread, cereal, etc. 1 serving vegetables; 1 serving fruit; 1 serving milk, yogurt, cheese; 2 servings fats, oils, sweets	About 700 calories	Tastes great. You are getting servings from 4 food groups. You have 35% of your calories if you are a female and 30% if you are a guy. So, guys, why not add another fruit if you want to increase your calories?

In addition to making good food choices, you need to think about food safety. We'll address food safety in more detail in Chapter 12, but you need to think about it if you're packing a lunch. Here are a few simple rules to follow:

- Keep cold foods cold so that bacteria don't grow.
  Use an insulated bag.
  Put an ice pack in the bag.

Table 11.6 The "Grab and Go" Lunch			
Food Item	**Pyramid**	**Calories**	**What's Good about It?**
Whole-wheat bagel, 1 ounce of red pepper hummus, 1 large apple, 8 ounces of nonfat chocolate milk	3 servings bread, 1 serving fruit, 1 serving dairy	603	Just grab and go. You are getting servings from 3 food groups. Really high in fiber.
Sesame seed bagel, 1 cup low-fat fruit yogurt, apple, 1% nonfat chocolate milk	3 servings bread, cereal, etc.; 1 serving fruit; 3 servings milk, yogurt, cheese; 10 servings fats, oils, sweets	Approximately 790	Just grab and go. You are getting servings from 3 food groups. You have 40% of your calories if you're a female and 35% if you're a male.

- Bacteria are more likely to grow in foods that are high in protein and water.
- Deli sandwiches, yogurt, cut fruit, and cheese all need to be kept cold.
- Keep hot food hot. Put soups, stews, and casserole-type items in a thermal container so that they maintain their temperature.

Following safe food-handling techniques can make a big difference. First, your food tastes better—that yogurt is cold and has better flavor and, better yet, you won't get sick. If you have any protein foods—deli meats, a piece of leftover chicken, or leftover pizza—you need to keep them cold. So make sure to put in an ice pack.

Eating Out

Some schools allow older students to go off-campus for lunch. If you go to one of the local food hangouts, just try to make good choices. Check out Chapter 9 on fast food. You can eat healthy at many of these places if you make educated choices, but if you do this daily, you'll need to make sure that your other meals provide any nutrition you don't get at lunch.

If you want to save some money on lunch, either choose the school lunch or brown-bag it. Eating out is the most expensive option. Usually, school meals are a good option financially, and you get a good nutritious meal. Bagging it is usually cheapest (because parents are really feeding you). The choice is yours.

SNACKING

Believe it or not, eating between meals is very important and should be done! You need to keep that engine running. Many kids today are very active and participate in sports. Practices are usually right after school, and you need some energy—fuel—in the form of calories to get you through that practice. So do yourself a favor and eat something before practice. You perform better if you have something in your stomach. Planning in advance helps. You can make better choices if you think in advance about what snacks are available.

Even if you're concerned with your calorie intake, snacking is okay. Many professionals feel that it is better for your metabolism if you eat more frequently. For more detail, read Chapter 5 on weight management. Basically, if you eat regularly, you are not starved at mealtime and therefore are less likely to overeat. Your body is more efficient if you are continually fueling it. Having a healthy snack can help curb your appetite and keep you going.

The key here is really healthy and nutritious snacks. It is not always easy to find good snacks. And you really don't want to fill up on junk foods and then not be hungry for a real meal that offers good nutrition. So what is good versus junk? There really is no food that is bad. Did we really say that? Yes, all foods can fit into a healthy diet. The issue is how much you eat and how frequently you eat it. It's a balancing act. There is nothing wrong with a candy bar. But several candy bars a day are just not a nutritious choice. See Table 11.7 for options.

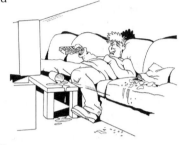

All of these items offer you something nutritious. What you need to think about is this: How much should I eat? When is my next meal? So watch your portions. Think about your activity level. Are you running, sitting in a club meeting, or texting? The more active you are, the more calories you need. The reverse is also true: the less active you are, the fewer calories you need.

Another time we snack is after dinner. Some of us eat early and need a boost to get through the evening. If you're falling asleep doing your homework, get up and have a snack. This should give you some energy to finish your work. Some of you might have a game or prac-tice after dinner and need a snack. You might want to think about not having dessert with dinner and saving it for a later snack. Don't forget about activity: If you're falling asleep doing your homework, you may benefit from a good round of jumping jacks.

DINNER

Lifestyles today have certainly changed the way we eat. We're eating out more than ever before. We're also bringing home more "take-out" food. There are a lot of single-parent households, families with two working parents, and active kids who need to be driven around to after-school activities. So where does that leave dinner? There's not enough time to prepare a meal, let alone eat at a reasonable hour together. It's great to have a family mealtime. This is an opportunity to catch up on what's happening with everyone. Unfortunately, with

Table 11.7 Ten Snacks to Consider		
Snack	Calories	What's Good about It?
Low-fat fruit yogurt	130	Good source of calcium.
1 ounce almonds	165	Good source of fiber and protein.
1 ounce pretzels	111	Good to grab. Good option if you want something salty.
1 ounce baked BBQ potato chips	120	Tastes great.
Chocolate chip Clif Bar	250	Good source of fiber and protein.
10 baby carrots and 2 tablespoons ranch dressing	180	Great crunch. Fabulous source of vitamin A.
5 saltines with 2 tablespoons peanut butter	318	Good source of protein; sticks with you.
Large apple	110	Tastes great and a fruit.
2 pieces of string cheese	160	Good source of protein and calcium.
Large banana	118	Easy to bring along and a fruit.

our busy lifestyles, for many families this just isn't possible on a nightly basis.

The meal principles discussed previously still apply here. Have about 33 percent of your day's calories at dinnertime. Make sure that you get foods from several of the different food groups on the food guide pyramid. At this meal, you really want to take a look at the vegetable group because this one may get ignored at other times during the day.

A Traditional Dinner

Entrée or main course: Protein food or vegetarian option
Side dishes:
    Starch: potatoes, rice, pasta, or bread
    Vegetable: salad or hot vegetable
Beverage: Milk or juice
Dessert: Fruit, pudding, or ice cream

What about that brownie sundae or apple pie? Nothing's wrong with sweet desserts, but see where you stack up for the day on the food guide pyramid. If you haven't had any or enough fruit, have fruit for dessert. Desserts often add fat and sugar, throwing your pyramid out of balance. But, once in a while, there is nothing wrong with just eating what you like. Enjoy!

QUICK MEALS TO MAKE AT HOME

There are lots of options in the grocery store to help you put together a quick and nutritious meal. Check out the freezer section. There are many new products that have vegetables, starches, and seasonings in them—all you need to do is add the meat, fish, or poultry. With many of these items, you are getting three of the food groups from the pyramid. There are also many boxed items like this. They are a great option for busy lifestyles. Remember that these items are usually more expensive because most of the preparation has been done for you. Also be aware that there is usually more sodium in these foods. But buying these packaged meals can still be less expensive than eating out. The choice is yours.

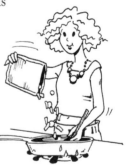

We have a few suggestions for some quick meals that you can put together in a hurry in Table 11.8. It's a good idea to take a look at the

Table 11.8 Quick Meals When You're in a Hurry	
Family Frittata	Make sure you have eggs, potatoes, green pepper, and onions in the pantry. Check out the recipe on page 206. Tastes great.
Pasta with Meat Sauce	Brown a pound of ground beef and add a jar of your favorite tomato sauce. Cook a pound of pasta, and dinner is served.
Braised Chicken with Tomatoes	A great quick recipe. Just have chicken thighs, onion, mustard, and a can of diced tomatoes. Cook some brown rice, and you're set for a delicious meal. Check out the recipe on page 198.
Egg and Cheese Tortilla Wrap	All alone? Scramble and cook a couple of eggs and a slice of American cheese and wrap it in a tortilla. Great quick meal.
Chicken and Stir Fry Vegetables	Leftover chicken. Stir fry some vegetables and add a little stir-fry sauce.

food label on the package to make sure that you'll get all the nutrition you need. In Chapter 11, you'll find detailed information about reading food labels.

QUICK MEALS TO PICK UP AND EAT AT HOME

Grocery stores have responded to customers' needs and now have sections that look like restaurants. They are usually located by the deli section and offer items such as roasted chicken, meatballs, stuffed fish, pastas, potatoes, vegetables, and salads. You can buy your entire meal. These are a huge trend in the food industry. Watch out, though. The more food is prepared by someone else for you, the more it costs. Nevertheless, this is still a much less expensive option than eating out. Make sure that you think about food safety when purchasing food this way.

Here are a few tips if you are purchasing prepared food:

- Look for cleanliness in the store where you are buying your food.
- Make sure that the food you're purchasing is properly refrigerated or frozen.
- Put refrigerated or frozen food in a refrigerator or freezer immediately when you get home.
- Don't make stops on the way home from the grocery store.
- Reheat cooked food to 165° F.

For more detail on food safety, check out Chapter 12.

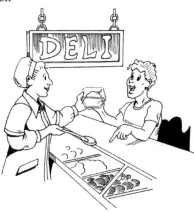

Another place for quick meals in the supermarket is the meat section. Not only are there chicken nuggets, but there is seasoned and cooked chicken ready to put in a salad or add to another dish. These are all great options for busy families. Just remember food safety. Reheat according to package directions. Make sure that the store you're purchasing from has safe food-handling procedures.

Fast-food restaurants have also responded to consumer demands. At some fast-food chains, you can pick up buckets, complete meals, whatever you want. If you live in an urban or suburban area, many restaurants will deliver to you. Families are feeling so rushed that they would like to eat at home, but they don't have the time or energy to do the preparation.

EATING OUT

So let's say you had a game, and it's late. Often, the quickest and easiest thing is to eat out. This might be a good time to review Chapter 9 on fast food. There are many restaurant options other than fast food. One of the biggest considerations if you're going to a restaurant is price. How much do you want to spend? Today there are restaurants that can fit into many different budgets. You just need to plan ahead.

Eating out at a restaurant with waiter or waitress service is not always a more nutritious option than fast food. You need to ask questions. Ask how the food item is prepared. If something is grilled, there is usually no extra fat being added to it. Is something served in a cream sauce? That means more fat.

If you are going out to a nice restaurant only occasionally, you needn't worry about what you're eating. But if you're going out several times a week, you may want to ask additional questions about how foods are prepared so that you're able to make better choices. Many restaurants identify food items that are healthier options. Some put a heart or an asterisk next to the menu item, indicating what they consider to be a better choice. Some chain restaurants are now putting calorie counts right on the menu. In addition, some states have passed laws requiring restaurants to tell customers the nutrition information for their menu items.

BALANCING YOUR CHOICES

Eating healthy can be fun and easy, but it does require some planning. The less you plan, the more likely you are to reach for quick, often less nutritious, options. Even though you can't expect to plan your menus every day, you can try to build a healthy diet overall and balance your choices.

When you reach for a snack or pack a lunch, take an extra second or two to think about your day. Could you make better choices? If you know you're going to a fast-food restaurant that evening, pack a leaner lunch with more fruits and vegetables because fast food can be limited in the fruit and vegetable choices. If you know you have an extra-long practice that day, pack an extra snack that is high in carbohydrates to get you through your workout feeling energetic. You really can have your cake and eat it, too—with a little planning. Balance your choices, and enjoy!

 There's an app for this, too. You can plan and rate your entire day of eating with an app. Download and start entering your meals. Check out the nutrition tips, quick snack apps, recipes and more.

KEY TERMS AND DEFINITIONS

National School Breakfast and Lunch programs: federally funded (by the U.S. Department of Agriculture) food programs developed to offer nutritious meals for children at school

Complete meal option: a meal sold as a unit (i.e., the entrée, side dishes, beverage, and dessert) as opposed to being sold à la carte

À la carte: food items that are sold as individual items; in the School Lunch Program, these items are not part of a complete lunch. Some examples are chips, cookies, and ice cream bars.

Cook It

L et's shop. Okay, so grocery shopping is not as much of a turn-on as clothes shopping or cruising the mall. But if you plan on doing any cooking, you've got to hit that grocery store. Let's see what you should think about before buying food.

There are many different kinds of shops where you can buy food: supermarkets; warehouse stores such as Sam's or Price Club; smaller grocery or specialty stores; convenience stores; and farm stands. Table 12.1 lists some things you may want to consider when deciding where to shop for food.

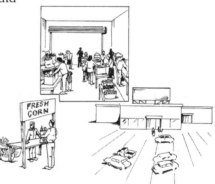

FOOD LABELS

Now that you've picked your store, you are ready to pick your food. To help you choose healthy foods when shopping, you should learn more about reading a food label. A lot of nutrition information is available on the food items that you purchase. Although most people refer to this as the food label, the real name is Nutrition Facts Label.

Table 12.1 A Comparison of Types of Stores	
Type of Store	**What Makes Them Different?**
Supermarkets	Have lots of items, good food selection. Usually have good prices, they're competitive. Are large so it might take some time to go through and find what you're looking for.
Warehouse stores	Great prices, but you usually need to purchase a large amount of an item—will you use it, or end up throwing it away? Often have a limited selection—you might not find everything you want, so you may need to go somewhere else.
Smaller grocery	Do not have as much of a selection as a supermarket or specialty store. Prices may be a little higher than a supermarket. Might be known for specific items, such as meat, produce, or ethnic foods.
Convenience stores	Have a very limited number of food items. Prices are usually expensive. Check expiration dates—because they don't have much inventory, they do not restock that often. Very convenient—sometimes the convenience is worth the price.
Farm stands	Fresh produce at great prices when the fruit or vegetables are in season. Locally grown produce tastes great. Try to use this whenever you can.

A federal regulation that came into effect in 1990 requires food companies to put nutrition information on food items in a specific manner. Figure 12.1 is an example of a food label with explanations of each section.

Let's take a closer look at some sections of the label:

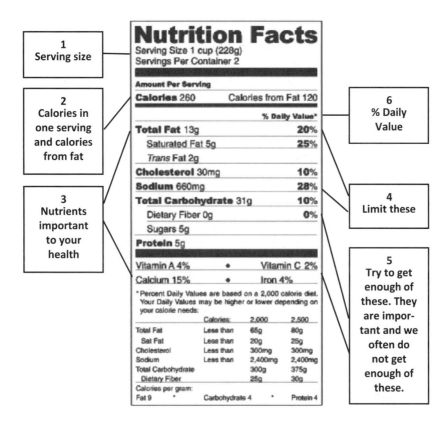

Figure 12.1 Example of a Food Label

1. Serving Size. This indicates what a normal serving size is of this food product and how many servings are in the container. Remember that if you eat a whole bag of chips and the label states there are 2 servings in the bag, you need to multiply everything by 2.

2. This line indicates calories for 1 serving and how many calories are from fat for this item.

3. This section lists nutrients that are important to your health and how much a serving of the food contributes to your daily intake, or % Daily Value. This section tells information about one serving.

4. The first nutrients listed are total fat, saturated fat, trans fats, cholesterol, and sodium. These are the items that you want to limit. Most Americans get enough of these. Eating too much of these might increase your risk of developing certain chronic diseases, such as heart disease, some cancers, and high blood pressure.

5. Dietary fiber, vitamins A and C, calcium, and iron are nutrients that most of us generally don't get enough of. You need to eat enough of these because they help prevent some diseases.

6. % of Daily Value (DV): These numbers tell us how 1 serving of this food fits into a 2,000 calorie diet. Depending on my many calories you need, this will vary. This is only a guide. The numbers you see do not add up to 100 percent. That is because the percentage you see for each nutrient relates to 100 percent of each nutrient. For example, if a label states that carbohydrate has a DV of 10 percent, you are getting 10 percent of the total carbohydrate that a "reference person" needs for the day. The label uses a reference person who is eating 2,000 calories/day.

You can see that there is a great deal of information in the grocery store. So take your time, and look at food labels. Interestingly, some items do not have to have a food label, such as fresh produce, meat, fish, and poultry. In the sections of the store where these food items are found, nutrition information should be available for your review. Ask the manager if you'd like to take a look at it.

Some products have particular terms on the label, such as light, reduced, and so on. The Food and Drug Administration (FDA) has specific rules that must be followed if certain words are used. The FDA is trying to make it easier on consumers to understand nutrition information and requires that products be labeled consistently. Table 12.2 explains some terms.

HEALTH CLAIMS

The FDA allows 12 health claims to be used on food products. These claims indicate a relationship between a nutrient or a food and the risk of a disease or health-related condition. Much research needs to

Table 12.2 Food Label Terms*	
Nutrient Content Claim	**What the Claim Means per Serving**
High (rich in, excellent source)	20% or more of the Daily Value
Good	10% to 19% of the Daily Value
More	Contains at least 10% more of the Daily Value for vitamins, minerals, protein, dietary fiber, or potassium.†
Light	Has at least one-third fewer calories or 50% less fat.† If more than half the calories are from fat, fat content must be reduced by 50% or more.
Less or fewer	Has 25% less of a nutrient or of calories
Calorie Claims	
Calorie-free	Less than 5 calories
Low-calorie	40 calories or less
Reduced calories	At least 25% fewer calories†
Sugar Claims	
Sugar-free	Less than 0.5 gram sugars
Reduced sugar	At least 25% less sugar†
Fiber Claims (If food is not low in total fat, the label must state total fat in conjunction with the fiber claims.)	
High fiber	5 grams or more

(continued on next page)

Table 12.2 Food Label Terms*	
Fiber Claims	**What the Claim Means per Serving**
Good source of fiber	2.5 grams to 4.9 grams
More or added fiber	At least 2.5 grams more†
Sodium Claims	
Sodium-free or salt-free	Less than 5 milligrams sodium
Very low sodium	35 milligrams of sodium or less
Low sodium	140 milligrams of sodium or less
Reduced sodium	At least 25% less sodium†
Light in sodium	At least 50% less sodium
Salt-free	Less than 5 milligrams sodium
Fat Claims	
Fat-free	Less than 0.5 gram fat
Low-fat	3 grams or less total fat
Reduced-fat	At least 25% less fat than the regular version
Saturated Fat Claims	
Saturated fat free	Less than 0.5 gram saturated fat and less than 0.5 gram trans fatty acids
Low in saturated fat	1 gram or less saturated fat and no more than 15% calories from saturated fat
Reduced saturated fat	At least 25% less saturated fat† and reduced by more than 1 gram fat
Note: Trans fat has no FDA-defined nutrient content claims.	

(continued on next page)

Table 12.2 Food Label Terms*	
Cholesterol Claims	
Cholesterol-free	Less than 2 milligrams cholesterol and 2 grams or less saturated fat
Low cholesterol	20 milligrams or less cholesterol and 2 grams or less saturated fat
Reduced cholesterol	At least 25% less cholesterol and 2 grams or less saturated fat†
Lean Claims	
Lean	Contains less than 10 grams total fat, 4.5 grams or less saturated fat, and less than 95 milligrams cholesterol
Extra lean	Contains less than 5 grams total fat, less than 2 grams saturated fat, and less than 95 milligrams cholesterol

* www.clemson.edu/extension/hgic/food/nutrition/nutrition/dietary_guide/hgic4061.html

† Compared to the reference (regular) food replaced.

be done before health claims are allowed. Table 12.3 outlines the current allowable health claims.

Ingredients that are contained in a food product are required to be listed on the label. The ingredients are listed in order by weight, from greatest to least.

Raw Fruits, Vegetables, and Fish

These foods need labeling but are not easy to label. You see many signs and posters in the departments in the store listing the nutrients for the most popular items.

Table 12.3 Health Claims the FDA Allows on Food Products	
Nutrient and Health Relationship	**Sample Claim on Manufacturer's Package**
Calcium and osteoporosis	"Regular exercise and a healthy diet with enough calcium helps teens and young adult white and Asian women maintain good bone health and may reduce their risk of osteoporosis in later life."
Dietary fat and cancer	"Development of cancer depends on many factors. A diet low in fat may reduce the risk of some cancers."
Fiber-containing grain products, fruits, and vegetables and cancer	"Low fat diets rich in fiber-containing grain products, fruits, and vegetables may reduce the risk of some types of cancer, a disease associated with many factors."
Fruits, vegetables and grain products that contain fiber, particularly soluble fiber, and risk of coronary heart disease	"Diets low in saturated fat and cholesterol and rich in fruits, vegetables, and grain products that contain some types of dietary fiber, particularly soluble fiber, may reduce the risk of heart disease, a disease associated with many factors."
Sodium and hypertension	"Diets low in sodium may reduce the risk of high blood pressure, a disease associated with many factors."
Fruits and vegetables and cancer	"Low fat diets rich in fruits and vegetables (foods that are low in fat and may contain dietary fiber, vitamin A, or vitamin C) may reduce the risk of some types of cancer, a disease associated with many factors. Broccoli is high in vitamins A and C, and it is a good source of dietary fiber."

(continued on next page)

Table 12.3 Health Claims the FDA Allows on Food Products	
Nutrient and Health Relationship	Sample Claim on Manufacturer's Package
Folate and neural tube defect	"Healthful diets with adequate folate may reduce a woman's risk of having a child with a brain or spinal cord defect."
Dietary noncariogenic carbohydrate sweeteners and dental caries	"Does not promote tooth decay."
Soluble fiber from certain foods and risk of coronary heart disease	"Soluble fiber from foods such as [name of soluble fiber source, and, if desired, name of food product], as part of a diet low in saturated fat and cholesterol, may reduce the risk of heart disease. A serving of [name of food product] supplies __ grams of the [necessary daily dietary intake for the benefit] soluble fiber from [name of soluble fiber source] necessary per day to have this effect."
Soy protein and risk of coronary heart disease	"Twenty-five grams of soy protein a day, as part of a low in saturated fat and cholesterol, may reduce the risk of heart disease. A serving of [name of food] supplies __ grams of soy protein."
Plant sterol and stanol esters and risk of coronary heart disease	"Foods containing at least 0.65 gram per of vegetable oil sterol esters, eaten twice a day with meals for a daily total intake of least 1.3 grams, as part of a diet low in saturated fat and cholesterol, may reduce the risk of heart disease. A serving of [name of food] supplies __ grams of vegetable oil sterol esters."

Food Allergy Information

Food allergies are a real problem, and the U.S. government has required labeling since 2006. Fish, milk, soybeans, wheat, eggs, shellfish, tree nuts, and peanuts are the most common food allergans and must be noted on the food package.

Front-of-Package Food Labeling

There has been lots of talk recently about food claims that are on the front of a food product. Food manufacturers started to put more nutritional information on the front of the package in addition to the nutrition facts label. Many grocery stores also began putting information on the shelves. Unfortunately, research has found that consumers may just look at these labels and not look at the whole picture that is given on the food label. Many consumers think some foods are better than they actually are.

As a result, the FDA is working with the USDA to ensure that all package labeling is consistent and not misleading to the consumer. They want the labeling to help consumers make healthy food choices.

Price Comparison

Beneath each food item in a store is a unit price. The unit price indicates how much a product costs for a unit of measurement. The price may be the cost of an item per ounce, for example. By looking at unit pricing, you are able to compare what is most cost-effective for you to purchase. You can compare different sized containers as well as different brands of a product.

When you are comparing prices, remember to think about how much you actually need. Just because it may be less expensive to buy a larger container, if you end up throwing some of the item away, it may not be worth it.

Expiration Dates

The federal government does not require expiration dates on foods, with the exception of infant formula and baby food. However, many states require that milk and other perishables be sold prior to an expiration date. The following are some terms that are commonly used when talking about expiration dates:

- Sell by _____. Don't buy the product after this date. This is the "expiration date."
- Best if used by _____. Flavor or quality is best by this date, but the product is still edible after the date stated.
- Use by _____. This is the last day that the manufacturer believes the product is of good quality. Foods are safe to eat if kept at 40°F or below, but be sure to follow the storage recommendations.

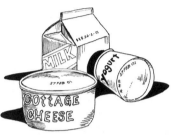

Shelf life is a common term used for food items. This term basically indicates how long the product is good to eat. Here is a guide for some perishable items:

Food and maximum storage period in refrigerator

Milk products: 5–7 days after the date on the container
Meat items, such as, chops, steaks, or roasts: 3–5 days after the date on the package
Ground meat: 1–2 days after the date on the package
Poultry and fish: 1–2 days after the date on the package
Fresh eggs: 3–5 weeks after you purchase them

These are guidelines, but remember that even if an item falls within these guidelines, if it doesn't smell or look good, it is best to throw it out.

New Trends

Changes are continually occurring in the food industry. We are hearing more about organic foods, and they certainly seem to be gaining in popularity. Not only are we seeing a growing section in produce departments of organic fruits and vegetables, but we are seeing more and more dairy and shelf-stable foods available as organic. "Organic" is a term that is regulated by the USDA. Figure 12.2 shows the organic labels that are allowed and explains the labeling standards.

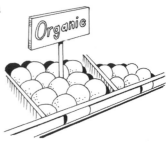

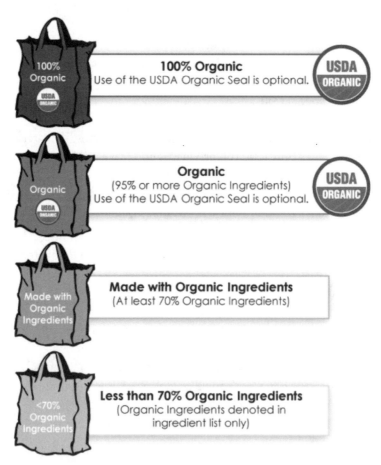

Figure 12.2. Organic Labeling

So let's take a look at what the term "organic" means. An organic food is one that is grown without using conventional pesticides and chemical fertilizers. For meat products, it means that the animals are fed organic feed and are given access to the outdoors. The animals are not fed antibiotics or growth hormones.

WHY CHOOSE ORGANIC?

People choose organic for different reasons. Some are concerned with the residues from chemicals and fertilizers and feel safer eating organic products. Other people are concerned with the impact of eating animals that have been fed antibiotics and hormones. Still others choose these products because of their positive impact on the environment.

IS ORGANIC WORTH IT?

You will find that organically grown food is more expensive. It also may not look as good as traditionally grown products. For example, an organically grown apple may not be as shiny and perfectly shaped, or a plum may not have the brightest color. We have no evidence that organic is nutritionally any better for you. It's simply a preference by the consumer. We find that many people choose to purchase some organic items and others traditionally grown. A nonprofit group called "The Environmental Working Group" has put together a list of what is termed "the dirty dozen and the clean fifteen." The dirty dozen are fruits and vegetables that have the highest amounts of pesticides, whereas the clean fifteen are foods with the least amount of pesticides. Check them out in Table 12.5. Notice that many of the clean fifteen have skins that you do not eat; as a result, these foods are not as affected by the pesticides. So if you are concerned about pesticide use, perhaps spend the extra money on the organic version for the items in the dirty dozen but buy the traditionally farmed clean fifteen.

Table 12.5 Pesticides in Produce	
The Dirty Dozen	**The Clean Fifteen**
celery	onion
peaches	avocado
strawberries	corn
apples	pineapple
blueberries	mangos
nectarines	sweet peas
bell peppers	asparagus
spinach	kiwi
kale	cabbage
cherries	eggplant
potatoes	cantaloupe
imported grapes	watermelon
	grapefruit
	sweet potatoes
	honeydew melon

You'll also see in the store that many items are labeled "natural." We know what organic means, but what does natural mean? Unfortunately, it doesn't really mean anything definite. The USDA has not come up with a definition of natural, so there are *no* standards. You should take a look at these products carefully and see if you want to spend any extra money on a product labeled as "natural."

"Sustainable agriculture" is a term we are hearing more and more. It sounds complicated, but it really just means being concerned about the environment and making a conscious effort to maintain our natural resources. That is why some people are trying to buy local food and produce whenever possible. This really helps the environment. Food production, packaging, and transportation produce carbon emissions, which have an impact on global warming. If you're interested in finding out more about how much carbon dioxide is produced from the foods you eat, check out a calculator at www.eatlowcarbon.org/#. The USDA has a program called "Know Your Farmer, Know Your Food." The goal is to get consumers in touch with what they eat. Local food often tastes better because it is fresher. It is most often sold at a better price too. So this trend really does seem to make sense. You'll notice when you buy local that the foods are available at different times, based on what is growing at that time.

Food shopping can be fun. Make a list so that you remember to purchase everything you need for the recipes you are making. You also want to make sure that you follow safe food-handling practices, the next topic.

SAFE FOOD HANDLING

Food safety is an important issue for everyone because we all eat food. If you are not careful with what foods you eat and drink, you can become very sick from foodborne diseases. Check out the food safety temperature guide. The danger zone is 40° to 140° (Figure 12.2). Food should be kept out of the danger zone as much as possible.

Here are some tips for safe food handling:

When Shopping
- Make a shopping list. Put all refrigerated and frozen foods at the end of the list. Put them in your shopping cart last so that they maintain a cool temperature.
- Check all expiration dates on the food labels (see specific details earlier in this chapter), and make sure that you will be using the food prior to that date.
- Make sure that all meat, fish, and poultry look and smell good. If in doubt, *do not buy*. Ground beef should be red, not brown.
- Put meat, fish, and poultry in a plastic bag so that juices do not leak onto other foods in your cart.
- Eggs should not be cracked or broken and should be grade A or AA.

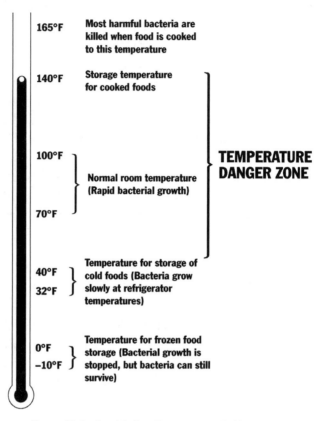

Figure 12.3   Food Safety Temperature Guide

- If you are purchasing any prepared food items, make sure that they are being stored under proper conditions—hot foods hot and cold foods cold.
- Make sure that you go home right away after grocery shopping, and put all items in the refrigerator or freezer immediately.

Storing Food
- The refrigerator should be at 40°F or below and the freezer at 0°F or below.
- Put raw meat, fish, and poultry on a dish before storing so that juices do not drip. Put these items on the lower shelves of the refrigerator.

Preparing Food
- Always wash hands in hot soapy water for 20 seconds, rubbing briskly. Rinse thoroughly, and dry hands with paper towel.
- Use separate cutting boards for produce and raw meat. If using just one, sanitize it after each use. Bacteria can be spread easily with cutting boards.
- Use cutting boards that can go in the dishwasher to be sanitized.
- Thaw food in the refrigerator, under running water at a temperature of 70°F or less, or in the microwave oven if you are cooking immediately after thawing.

Cooking Food
- Cook foods to the proper temperature (in degrees Fahrenheit)

Poultry	165°
Beef , rare	145°
Beef, medium	160°
Beef, well-done	170°
Ground beef	160°
Pork	160°
Eggs	160°
Casseroles	165°
Leftovers	165°

- All cooked food should be kept at 140°F or above after cooking.
- Cook eggs until the yolks and whites are firm, not runny.
- Do not eat raw eggs.
- Wash hands frequently during food preparation. Always wash hands after handling raw meats, fish, and poultry.
- Never put cooked food on a dish that was holding raw meat, fish, or poultry.
- Wash knives and other utensils after they have come in contact with raw meat, fish, or poultry.

Serving and Storing Food
- Always use clean dishes and utensils.

- Never leave food on the counter to cool. Put leftovers in the refrigerator immediately. Put leftovers in containers that can be properly closed.
- Use leftovers within 3 to 5 days.
- If you freeze leftovers, put in serving-size containers so that you are able to defrost properly. Use food items within 2 months.

OUR RECIPES AND UNDERSTANDING NUTRIENT ANALYSIS

A recipe contest was held in the state of Connecticut when we wrote the first edition of this book. The contest was advertised to teachers in middle and high schools and to school food service directors. Many people, especially students and teachers, submitted a variety of recipes. All recipes were tested and evaluated for quality in the Foods Laboratory at the University of Connecticut, Department of Nutritional Sciences. The best recipes were selected to include in this book. These are great recipes, and we want to share them with you. We have added a few more to round out the collection.

Each recipe has been analyzed for several nutrients. When completing nutrient analysis, the following guidelines were used:

- If more than one ingredient is listed, the first one that appears is used for nutrient analysis. For example, if butter or margarine is an option, butter is used for analysis.
- If a range is given for a recipe—for example, 1½ to 2 cups—the first amount given is used.

When looking at the nutrients for a recipe, don't look at just one item—look at your intake of all the nutrients over the whole day or several days.

We have also analyzed how each recipe fits into the food guide pyramid. Using the same methods as stated for nutrient analysis, we computed how many servings of each food group are met by eating 1 serving of the recipe. The information was rounded to the nearest whole or half number for a serving in each food group. We shortened the names of the food groups for ease in reading, as follows:

Bread, cereal, rice, and pasta group: Grain group
Vegetable group: Vegetable group
Fruit group: Fruit group
Meat poultry, fish, dry beans, eggs, and nuts group: Meat group
Milk, yogurt, and cereal group: Milk group
Fats, oils, and sweets: Fats, oils, and sweets

Take a look at the recipes and give some a try. Hope you enjoy them!

RECIPES

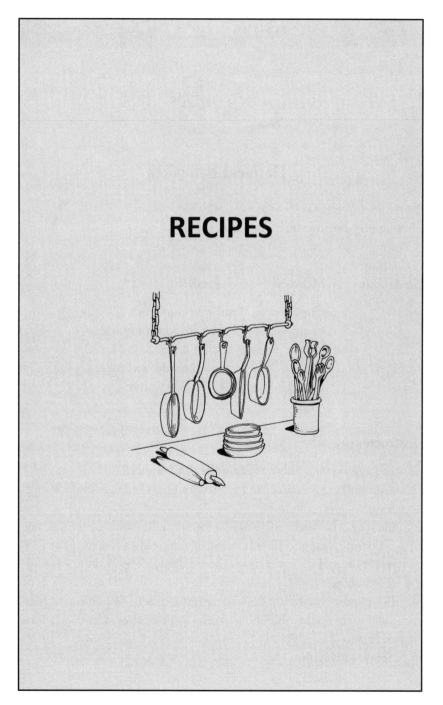

BREAKFAST

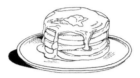

Oatmeal Pancakes

Serving: 4 (3 each)
Active preparation time: 10 minutes
Cooking time: 8 minutes to cook all pancakes

Amount	Measure	Ingredient
1¼	Cups	all-purpose flour
½	Cup	old-fashioned or quick oats
1	Cup	nonfat milk
½	Cup	applesauce, unsweetened
1	Each	egg, lightly beaten
½	Cup	pancake syrup

Instructions:

1. In large bowl, combine flour and oats. Mix well.
2. Add milk, applesauce, and egg to dry ingredients. Mix until moistened. Do not overmix.
3. Heat griddle over medium heat. Spray skillet with cooking spray. To ensure that griddle is hot enough, sprinkle a few drops of water on it. The water drops should dance. The griddle is ready for cooking.
4. Pour approximately ¼ cup batter onto griddle. When top of pancake is covered with bubbles, turn to cook other side. (Only turn over once.)
5. Serve with syrup.

Oats are a super grain, not just good for breakfast; try for a quick supper.

Nutrient Analysis (per serving): 354 calories, 8% calories from fat, 2% calories from saturated fat, iron 3 mg, vitamin C 1 mg, vitamin A 59 µg, calcium 94 mg, fiber 2 g.

Food Guide Pyramid: 2 ounces grain.

Banana Bran Muffins

Servings: 12 muffins
Oven temperature: 375°
Cooking time: 15–20 minutes

Amount	Measure	Ingredient
1	cup	all-purpose flour
1	cup	wheat bran
1	teaspoon	baking soda
½	teaspoon	salt
½	cup	walnuts or pecans
1	cup	ripe banana, mashed
½	cup	butter, unsalted, softened
1	medium	egg
½	cup	brown sugar

Instructions:

1. Preheat oven to 375°.
2. Grease muffin pans or use cupcake papers.
3. Stir together flour, wheat bran, baking soda, salt, and nuts.
4. In another bowl, beat together banana and butter until well blended.
5. Add egg and brown sugar to banana mixture, and beat until completely mixed.
6. Add dry ingredients to banana mixture, and stir until just blended. Do not overmix.
7. Spoon into muffin pans.
8. Bake for 15–20 minutes until toothpick inserted in center comes out clean. Let cool for 5 minutes before removing from pan.

Good for breakfast or a snack. Contains the superfood nuts.

Nutrient Analysis (per serving): 205 calories, 48% calories from fat, 22% from saturated fat, iron 1 mg, vitamin C 2 mg, vitamin A 101 µg, calcium 19 mg, fiber 3 g

Food Guide Pyramid: 1 ounce grain; 3 teaspoons fats, oils, and sweets.

Recipe submitted by Matt Stefanelli while attending Waterford High School, Waterford, CT.

Breakfast Burrito Wrap

Servings: 8 each
Cooking time: 15 minutes

Amount	Measure	Ingredient
8	slices	turkey bacon
1	medium	onion, chopped
1	medium	red pepper, chopped
9	large	eggs (or 2 cups egg substitute)
8	8 inch	flour tortillas
1	cup	Monterey jack cheese
(reduced fat optional)		

Instructions:

1. Fry bacon in nonstick frying pan, drain and crumble bacon, set aside.
2. In same pan, cook onions and red pepper until tender, about 5 minutes.
3. Remove and set aside.
4. Warm tortillas in oven or microwave.
5. Cook eggs in nonstick skillet over medium heat without stirring, until eggs begin to set.
6. Stir eggs gently and allow eggs to set until cooked through.
7. Add bacon and vegetables to eggs.
8. Spoon mixture onto tortillas, top with cheese.
9. Fold or roll tortillas.

Top with salsa if you like.

Red pepper is a good source of vitamins A and C.
Great for a quick lunch or supper.

Nutrient Analysis (per serving): 294 calories, 49% calories from fat, 9% from saturated fat, iron 1 mg, vitamin C 37 mg, vitamin A 453 µg, calcium 145 mg, fiber 3 g.

Food Guide Pyramid: ½ ounce grain; 1/3 cup vegetable; 1 ounce meat; ½ cup milk; 1 teaspoon fats, oils, and sweets.

Recipe submitted by Chris McLaughlin while attending Region District #5, Bethany, CT.

BEVERAGES

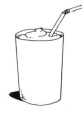

Angel-Devil Smoothie

Servings: 4

Amount	Measure	Ingredient
2	cups	vanilla yogurt, fat-free
2	cups	frozen strawberries, sliced
2		nonfat chocolate cookies or nonfat brownies
¼	cup	fat-free (skim) milk

Instructions:

1. Combine all ingredients in blender or food processor.
2. Pulse until mixture is pureed.
3. Serve immediately.

Great source of calcium and contains two super foods: yogurt and berries.

Nutrient Analysis (per serving): 196 calories, 1% calories from fat, 0% from saturated fat, iron 1 mg, vitamin C 53 mg, vitamin A 56 µg, calcium 186 mg, fiber 3 g.

Food Guide Pyramid: ½ ounce grain; 1 cup fruit; ½ cup milk ; 6 teaspoons fats, oils, and sweets.

Recipe submitted by Cindy Connor, RD, Milbrook, NY.

Banana Shake

Servings: 2

Amount	Measure	Ingredient
1	cup	vanilla soy milk beverage, chilled
5	ounces	silken tofu, chilled and cubed
2	cups	banana, fresh or frozen
1½	tablespoons	honey
½	teaspoon	vanilla extract

Instructions:

1. Combine all ingredients in a blender.
2. Blend until smooth.

Low-fat smoothie with the superfood soy.
Great vegetarian option for breakfast, snack, or dessert.

Nutrient Analysis (per serving): 320.9 calories, 12% calories from fat, 3% from saturated fat, iron 2 mg, vitamin C 14 mg, vitamin A 37 µg, calcium 72 mg, fiber 4 g.

Food Guide Pyramid: 1½ servings fruit ; ½ cup milk; 3 servings fats, oils, and sweets.

Recipe submitted by Britain Vitale and Casey Yaglowski while attending Regional District #17, Higganum, CT.

Fruit Concoction

Servings: 6 (6-ounce servings)

Amount	Measure	Ingredient
4–5	medium	ice cubes
2½	cups	orange juice
1	medium	banana
10	medium	strawberries, fresh or frozen
½	cup	vanilla yogurt or soy yogurt
2	teaspoons	honey
2	teaspoons	wheat germ

Instructions:

1. Put ice cubes in blender with 1¼ cups orange juice, banana, and strawberries.
2. Add yogurt, honey, and wheat germ.
3. Blend until smooth and frothy.
4. Add remaining 1¼ cups of orange juice.
5. Blend until desired smoothness.

A low-fat smoothie— and it's a fruit too.

Nutrient Analysis (per serving): 95 calories, 8% calories from fat, 4% from saturated fat, iron 0 mg, vitamin C 25 mg, vitamin A 14 µg, calcium 44 mg, fiber 1 g.

Food Guide Pyramid: 1 cup fruit; 1 teaspoon fats, oils, and sweets.

Recipe submitted by Don Walkwitz, teacher, Conard High School, West Hartford, CT.

SOUPS, STEWS, AND SIDES

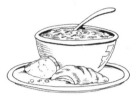

Barley and Mushroom Risotto

Servings: 8

Amount	Measure	Ingredient
6½	cups	low-fat chicken broth
¼	cup	olive oil
1		medium onion, chopped
3	cloves	garlic, minced
2	cups	pearl barley
10	ounces	mushrooms, sliced
½	cup	parmesan cheese

Instructions:

1. Bring broth to a simmer and keep warm.
2. In medium pan, heat olive oil. Add chopped onion and garlic; sauté until tender.
3. Add barley to onion mixture and cook to coat barley with the olive oil. Add mushrooms and sauté about 5 minutes.
4. Add 1 cup of warm broth, stir and cook until water is absorbed. Continue adding broth and cooking until absorbed. This takes about 45 minutes.
5. When barley is tender, turn off heat and add parmesan cheese and serve.

Barley is a super grain. Great with grilled chicken.

Continued on next page

Nutrient Analysis (per serving): 263 calories, 15% calories from fat, 11% from saturated fat, iron 2 mg, vitamin C 1 mg, vitamin A 3 µg, calcium 25 mg, fiber 9 g.

Food Guide Pyramid: 2 ounces grain; ½ cup vegetable; 1 1/3 teaspoon fats, oils, and sweets.

Broccoli Slaw

Servings: 6

Amount	Measure	Ingredient
½	12-ounce package	broccoli coleslaw
½	cup	dry roasted sunflower seeds
½	cup	golden raisins
2	tablespoons	sliced almonds

Dressing:

3	tablespoons	canola oil
2	tablespoons	cider vinegar
2	tablespoons	sugar
½	packet	beef ramen seasoning packet
1	package	beef ramen noodles

Instructions:

1. Mix broccoli coleslaw, sunflower seeds, raisins, and almonds in large bowl.
2. Combine ingredients for dressing. Whisk well.
3. Pour dressing on vegetable mixture and mix to combine.
4. Prior to serving, crumble ramen noodles over slaw and mix to combine. Serve immediately.

Broccoli is a super veggie. Most teens love the crunch.

Nutrient Analysis (per serving): 264 calories, 23% calories from fat, 6% calories from saturated fat, vitamin A 78 µg, vitamin C 53 mg, iron 2 mg, calcium 53 mg, fiber 3 g.

Food Guide Pyramid: ¾ cup vegetable; ½ ounce meat; ¾ cup fruit; 3 teaspoons fats, oils, and sweets.

Recipe by Colleen Thompson, MS, RD.

David's Three-Alarm Chili

Servings: 8
Cooking time: 1½ hours

Amount	Measure	Ingredient
1	pound	lean ground beef
3	15-ounce cans	red or pink kidney beans, drained
2	large	onions, chopped
3	large	green bell peppers, chopped
1	medium	garlic clove, minced
2	28-ounce cans	crushed tomatoes
3	tablespoons	chili powder
1	tablespoon	hot sauce
		cheddar cheese, shredded (optional)

Instructions:

1. Cook ground beef in large saucepan until well done. Drain fat.
2. Add beans, onions, peppers, and garlic to meat.
3. Add tomatoes, chili powder, and hot sauce to saucepan.
4. Simmer for 1½ hours on medium-low heat.
5. Adjust chili powder to taste.

Serving suggestion: Serve with shredded cheddar cheese and corn bread.

Great source of fiber and vitamin A. Beans are a superfood too.

Nutrient Analysis (per serving): 351 calories, 20% calories from fat, 7% from saturated fat, iron 7 mg, vitamin C 67 mg, vitamin A 809 µg, calcium 135 mg, fiber 17 g.

Food Guide Pyramid: 5½ servings vegetable; 1 serving meat.

Recipe submitted by David Nettleton while attending Bunnell High School, Stratford, CT.

Geoff's Corn and Bean Chowder

Servings: 10
Cooking time: 30–40 minutes

Amount	Measure	Ingredient
1	15½-ounce can	corn
1	19-ounce can	black beans
1	15-ounce can	garbanzo beans
1	15½-ounce can	red kidney beans
2	tablespoons	oil
4	cloves	garlic, minced
2	medium	onions, chopped
4	cups	vegetable or chicken broth
2	8-ounce cans	tomato sauce
½	teaspoon	oregano (can add more to taste)
½	teaspoon	sweet basil (can add more to taste)
		salt (optional) to taste
		pepper (optional) to taste
1	12-ounce can	evaporated milk

Instructions:

1. Drain corn and beans. Set aside.
2. Heat oil in soup pot. Sauté onion and garlic until tender.
3. Add beans, corn, broth, tomato sauce, and spices.
4. Bring to boil and then simmer 30–40 minutes.
5. Remove small amount from pot and gradually add evaporated milk. Slowly pour into soup pot. Do not boil or milk will curdle.

Great source of fiber. Contains beans, a superfood.

Continued on next page

Nutrient Analysis (per serving): 274 calories, 22% calories from fat, 5% from saturated fat, iron 3 mg, vitamin C 6 mg, vitamin A 72 µg, calcium 137 mg, fiber 11 g.

Food Guide Pyramid: 1½ servings vegetable; ½ serving meat; 1 serving milk.

Recipe submitted by Kathy Tucker, parent, Clinton, CT.

Quinoa and Black Bean Salad

Servings: 12

Amount	Measure	Ingredient
3	cups	quinoa, dry
1	15-ounce can	black beans, drained and rinsed
1	medium	red bell pepper, chopped
2	cups	corn kernels, fresh or frozen
3	tablespoons	parsley, chopped
1½	tablespoons	basil, dried
½	cup	extra virgin olive oil
½	cup	red wine vinegar
1	teaspoon	Dijon mustard

Instructions:

1. Prepare quinoa according to package directions (rinse, drain, cook).
2. Combine cooked quinoa with black beans, chopped pepper, corn, parsley, and basil. Mix well.
3. Make dressing: whisk olive oil, red wine vinegar, and Dijon mustard.
4. Add dressing to quinoa mixture.

Quinoa tastes great and is a superfood; give it a try.

Nutrient Analysis (per serving): 263 calories, 18% calories from fat, 7% from saturated fat, iron 4 mg, vitamin C 21 mg, vitamin A 94 µg, calcium 27 mg, fiber 6 g.

Food Guide Pyramid: 2½ ounces grain; 1¾ teaspoons fats, oils, and sweets.

Recipe by Dana Angelo White, RD

Tortellini Salad

Servings: 18
Cooking time: 10 minutes

Amount	Measure	Ingredient
1	cup	rotelle noodles
8	ounces	cheese tortellini, fresh or frozen
2	medium	tomatoes
2	crowns	broccoli
½	6-ounce can	pitted black olives
1	small	red onion
¼	pound	Monterey jack cheese, unsliced
¼	pound	pepperoni, unsliced
1	16-ounce bottle	Italian salad dressing

Instructions:

1. Boil 2/3 quarts of water in one pot. Add rotelle and cook until tender.
2. Drain and let pasta cool for 8–10 minutes.
3. Boil 2 quarts of water in another pot. Add tortellini and simmer for 8 minutes on medium heat.
4. Drain and set tortellini aside to cool.
5. Chop tomatoes and cut up broccoli.
6. Slice olives and onion.
7. Cube cheese and cut up pepperoni.
8. Combine pasta with previous ingredients and salad dressing. Mix well.

If you'd like to lower the fat, try low-fat or fat-free dressing.

Nutrient Analysis (per serving): 207 calories, 72% calories from fat, 13% from saturated fat, iron 1 mg, vitamin C 11 mg, vitamin A 65 μg, calcium 45 mg, fiber 1 g.

Food Guide Pyramid: ½ serving grain; ½ serving vegetable; 1 serving fats, oils, and sweets.

Recipe submitted by Jennifer Lapkowski while attending Waterford High School, Waterford, CT.

ENTREES

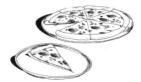

Wrestler's Low-Fat Low-Cal Garden Veggie Soup

Servings: approx. 6
Cooking time: 35 minutes

Amount	Measure	Ingredient
2	medium	celery stalks, chopped
1	large	onion, chopped
2	medium	carrots, chopped
1	medium	white potato, diced
2	14½-ounce cans	chicken broth, fat-free or low sodium
1	14½-ounce can	green beans, drained
1	10-ounce package	frozen spinach, thawed
1	14½-ounce can	stewed tomatoes, Italian-style
1/8	cup	fresh parsley
1	teaspoon	ground sage
2	envelopes	instant chicken broth, low-sodium
		parmesan cheese garnish (optional)

Instructions:

1. Combine all ingredients in large saucepan and bring to boil.
2. Reduce heat to low and simmer covered until vegetables are tender, approximately 30 minutes.
3. Serve with parmesan cheese if desired.

Good source of vitamins A and C and fiber.

Nutrient Analysis (per serving): 100 calories, 3% calories from fat, 0% from saturated fat, iron 4 mg, vitamin C 35 mg, vitamin A 3340 µg, calcium 127 mg, fiber 6 g.

Food Guide Pyramid: 4 cups vegetable.

Recipe submitted by Nick Poirier while attending Waterford High School, Waterford, CT.

Braised Chicken with Tomatoes

Servings: 4

Amount	Measure	Ingredient
8	each	chicken thighs, boneless and skinless
¼	cup	flour
¼	cup	olive oil
1	medium	onion, chopped
3	cloves	garlic, chopped
½	cup	cooking wine
3	tablespoons	Dijon mustard
½	cup	water
1	14½-ounce can	diced tomatoes

Instructions:

1. Coat chicken with flour.
2. In a 5-quart pan with a tight fitting lid, heat olive oil. Add chicken thighs and brown. Remove chicken thighs to a plate when browned.
3. Add onion and garlic and sauté until tender. Add cooking wine, mustard, and water. Bring to a boil. Add diced tomatoes and heat.
4. Return chicken thighs to pan. Cover and simmer until chicken is tender, about 30 minutes.

Tastes great. Looks fancy but really easy to prepare.

Nutrient Analysis (per serving): 424 calories, 38% calories from fat, 25% from saturated fat, iron 3 mg, vitamin C 15 mg, vitamin A 71 μg, calcium 75 mg, fiber 1 g.

Food Guide Pyramid: ½ cups vegetable; 4 ounces meat; 3 teaspoons fats, oils, and sweets.

Recipe by Ellen Shanley, MBA, RD, CD-N

Chicken Tacos

Servings: 9 (2 tacos per serving)
Oven temperature: 350°
Cooking time: 5–7 minutes

Amount	Measure	Ingredient
18	each	corn taco shells (hard)
1¼	pounds	ground chicken
1	16-ounce can	refried beans
1	1¼ envelopes	taco seasoning mix
1	8-ounce package	pre-mixed taco cheese
1	medium	head iceberg lettuce, shredded
2	large	tomatoes, chopped
1	cup	salsa

Instructions:

1. Preheat oven to 350°.
2. Brown ground chicken and drain fat.
3. Add taco seasoning mix according to package directions.
4. Add refried beans to chicken.
5. Divide chicken mixture among taco shells.
6. Sprinkle cheese on tacos.
7. Bake for 5–7 minutes or until cheese melts.
8. Add toppings of lettuce, tomatoes, and salsa.

Great source of fiber, vitamin A, and calcium.

Continued on next page

Nutrient Analysis (per serving): 516 calories, 30% calories from fat, 13% from saturated fat, iron 4 mg, vitamin C 21 mg, vitamin A 354 µg, calcium 227 mg, fiber 12 g.

Food Guide Pyramid: 1 ounce grain; 1 cup vegetable; ½ cup milk.

Recipe submitted by Sarah Houlihan while attending Waterford High School, Waterford, CT.

Chili-Cornmeal Skillet Pie

Servings: 4
Oven temperature: 350°
Cooking time: ~60 minutes

Amount	Measure	Ingredient
½	tablespoon	olive oil
1½	pounds	ground beef, 85% lean
1	medium	onion, chopped
1	medium	green bell pepper, chopped
1	tablespoon	chili powder
1	teaspoon	minced garlic
1	15-ounce can	kidney beans
1	8-ounce can	tomato sauce
		cornmeal mush (recipe follows)

Instructions:

1. Preheat oven to 350° degrees.
2. Heat oil in large ovenproof skillet over medium heat.
3. Add beef, onion, bell pepper, chili powder, and garlic.
4. Sauté until vegetables are tender and beef is no longer pink, breaking up beef with back of spoon, about 10 minutes.
5. Add drained beans and tomato sauce. Simmer until chili is slightly thickened and beef is cooked through, about 10 minutes.
6. Spoon cornmeal mush over chili, covering completely.
7. Place skillet in oven and bake until topping is golden brown and chili is bubbling at edges, about 40 minutes.
8. Let pie stand for 10 minutes.
9. Spoon onto plates and serve.

Great fiber source.

Continued on next page

Nutrient Analysis (per serving): 365 calories, 27% calories from fat, 9% from saturated fat, iron 4 mg, vitamin C 26 mg, vitamin A 145 μg, calcium 50 mg, fiber 9 g.

Food Guide Pyramid: 2 ounces grain; ¾ cup vegetable; 2 ounces meat.

Cornmeal Mush

Active preparation time: 30 minutes
Cooking time: ~60 minutes

Amount	Measure	Ingredient
1	cup	yellow cornmeal
1	tablespoon	sugar
½	teaspoon	salt
¼	teaspoon	pepper
1	15-ounce can	whole kernel corn, drained, liquid reserved
2	each	eggs, large

Instructions:

1. Preheat oven to 350° degrees.
2. Combine cornmeal, sugar, salt, and pepper in heavy large saucepan.
3. Pour reserved corn liquid into large measuring cup. Add enough water to measure 2¾ cups.
4. Whisk liquid mixture into cornmeal. Add corn.
5. Using wooden spoon, stir over medium-high heat until mixture is thick and begins to boil, about 10 minutes.
6. Cool to lukewarm, stirring occasionally, about 15 minutes.
7. Mix in eggs, spread in on top of Chili-Cornmeal Skillet Pie or place in buttered 10-inch diameter pie plate.
8. Bake cornmeal mixture until firm to touch, about 40 minutes.
9. Let stand 10 minutes. Cut into wedges.

Easy Pizza

Servings: 6
Oven temperature: 450°
Cooking time: 8–10 minutes

Amount	Measure	Ingredient
1½	cups	all-purpose baking mix
1/3	cup	hot water
1	8-ounce jar	pizza sauce
2	ounces	sliced pepperoni
2	slices	bacon, cooked and chopped
¼	cup	mushrooms, sliced
¼	cup	green pepper, chopped
¼	cup	onion, chopped
3	ounces	mozzarella cheese, shredded

Instructions:

1. Preheat oven to 450° and grease cookie sheet.
2. Place baking mix and water in small bowl and stir with fork until soft dough forms.
3. Flatten dough with hands and sprinkle small amount of flour on each side.
4. Roll dough onto cookie sheet using rolling pin.
5. Top dough with pizza sauce, toppings, and cheese.
6. Bake 8–10 minutes, until cheese bubbles.

If you don't like these vegetables, add whatever vegetables you like.

Nutrient Analysis (per serving): 280 calories, 50% calories from fat, 19% from saturated fat, iron 2 mg, vitamin C 11 mg, vitamin A 141 µg, calcium 124 mg, fiber 2 g.

Food Guide Pyramid: 1 ounce grain; 1 cup vegetable; ½ ounce meat; ½ cup milk; ½ teaspoon fats, oils, and sweets.

Recipe submitted by Marilyn Schwab, teacher, Fair Haven Middle School, New Haven, CT.

Family Frittata

Serving: 4
Cooking time: 35 minutes

Amount	Measure	Ingredient
1	teaspoon	olive oil
		cooking spray
½	cup	onion, chopped
½	cup	green bell pepper, chopped
1	pound	potatoes, sliced, leave skin on
¾	teaspoon	salt
¼	teaspoon	black pepper
4	large	eggs
2	tablespoons	dried parsley
4	tablespoons	salsa

Instructions:

1. Heat oil in a 10-inch nonstick skillet coated with cooking spray over medium heat. Add onion and bell pepper; sauté for 5 minutes until vegetables are tender.
2. Arrange potatoes over onion mixture; sprinkle with salt and black pepper.
3. Cover and reduce heat to medium low. Cook for 20 minutes or until potatoes are tender.
4. Preheat broiler.
5. Combine eggs and parsley in a medium bowl. Whisk until well combined. Pour over vegetables.
6. Cook over medium heat for 10 minutes or until almost set. Cover skillet so that eggs cook through. Remove from heat and broil until browned and set.
7. Cut into wedges and top with salsa.

Eggs are superfood. If you want to take even less time in preparation, microwave the potatoes for about 3 minutes and then slice. They will be precooked and will not take the same amount of cooking time.

Nutrient Analysis (per serving): 233 calories, 25% calories from fat, 7% from saturated fat, iron 3 mg, vitamin C 32 mg, vitamin A 108 µg, calcium 55 mg, fiber 0 g.

Food Guide Pyramid: ½ cup vegetable; 1 ounce meat.

Mexican Veggie Wrap

Servings: 6
Oven temperature: 350°
Cooking time: 30 minutes

Amount	Measure	Ingredient
1	tablespoon	oil
1	cup	broccoli florets
1	medium	red bell pepper, cut into strips
1	medium	zucchini, sliced thin
1	medium	carrot, shredded
2	cups	cabbage, shredded
1	12-ounce jar	salsa
1½	cups	Monterey jack cheese, shredded
6	8-inch	flour tortillas

Instructions:

1. Preheat oven to 350°.
2. Heat oil in skillet. Sauté vegetables in oil until tender.
3. Add salsa and cook an additional 10 minutes.
4. Remove from heat and stir in ¾ cup of the cheese.
5. Place flour tortillas on a cookie sheet.
6. Spoon mixture evenly onto each tortilla.
7. Close tortilla by wrapping or rolling. Place in baking dish.
8. Sprinkle with remaining cheese.
9. Bake for 20 minutes or until cheese is melted.

Broccoli is a super veggie. Broccoli, peppers, and carrots are great sources of vitamins A and C.

Nutrient Analysis (per serving): 305 calories, 44% calories from fat, 18% from saturated fat, iron 3 mg, vitamin C 78 mg, vitamin A 1,464 μg, calcium 311 mg, fiber 3 g.

Food Guide Pyramid: 1½ ounces grain; 2 cups vegetable; ½ cup milk.

Recipe submitted by Betsey Perkins, teacher, Central High School, Bridgeport, CT.

Pasta and Beans

Servings: 4
Cooking time: 30 minutes

Amount	Measure	Ingredient
2	tablespoons	olive oil
1	large	onion, chopped
2	cloves	garlic, minced
1	cup	tomato sauce
½	cup	tomato paste
3	cups	water
1	teaspoon	salt
½	teaspoon	pepper
¼	teaspoon	crushed red pepper flakes
1	15½-ounce can	red kidney beans, drained
1	15½-ounce can	cannellini beans(white beans), drained
1	8½-ounce can	green peas, drained
½	pound	ditalini (tiny tubular pasta), cooked according to package parmesan cheese, (optional)

Instructions:

1. Heat oil in large pan. Sauté onion and garlic until tender.
2. Add tomato sauce, tomato paste, and water.
3. Add salt, pepper, and red pepper flakes.
4. Bring to a boil and simmer 15 minutes.
5. Add beans, peas, and cooked ditalini. Add parmesan cheese to taste.

Great vegetarian meal with lots of fiber.

Nutrient Analysis (per serving): 43 calories, 17% calories from fat, 2% from saturated fat, iron 5 mg, vitamin C 15 mg, vitamin A 349 µg, calcium 92 mg, fiber 16 g.

Food Guide Pyramid: 1½ ounces grain; 2 cups vegetable; ½ ounce meat; ½ teaspoon fats, oils, and sweets.

Recipe submitted by Lori Koladicz while attending Silas Deane Middle School, Wethersfield, CT.

Pasta with Chicken and Broccoli

Serving: 4
Cooking time: 30 minutes

Amount	Measure	Ingredient
12	ounces	fettuccini pasta
1½	cup	broccoli, chopped
1½	cup	chicken, shredded
1	tablespoon	butter
1/3	cup	parmesan cheese
Lemon sauce:		
1¼	cup	cooking wine
¾	cup	chicken broth, low-fat and low-sodium
3	tablespoons	lemon juice
1	tablespoons	oregano, dried

Instructions:

1. Boil fettuccini according to package directions.
2. While fettuccini is cooking, make lemon sauce. Put cooking wine into a small saucepan. Bring to a boil and cook until reduced by a fourth, approximately 5 minutes. Add broth, lemon juice, and oregano. Bring to a boil and reduce to one-fourth. You will have about 1½ cups of sauce.
3. Put broccoli in a microwave safe bowl and microwave for 3 minutes.
4. Drain fettuccini. Put lemon sauce, chicken, and broccoli in large pot and heat through. Stir in butter.
5. Add drained pasta and parmesan cheese. Mix thoroughly.

Tastes great and has a super veggie: broccoli.

Nutrient Analysis (per serving): 510.0 calories, 14.5% calories from fat, 21.8% from saturated fat, iron 2.7 mg, vitamin C 22.2 mg, vitamin A 94.9 μg, calcium 27.6 mg, fiber 1.5 g.

Food Guide Pyramid: 4 ounces grain; 1 ounce meat; ½ teaspoon fats, oils, and sweets.

Recipe submitted by Tina Twiggs, teacher, Sheehan High School, Wallingford, CT.

Penne with Tomatoes and Chicken

Servings: 4
Oven temperature: 350°
Cooking time: 30–40 minutes

Amount	Measure	Ingredients
¼	cup	tomatoes, chopped
½	cup	boiling water
6	ounces	boneless chicken breast
¼	cup	white cooking wine
1	tablespoon	Italian seasoning
2	medium	garlic cloves, minced
8	ounces	penne
1	tablespoon	flour
1	12-ounce can	evaporated milk
		cooking spray

Instructions:

1. Preheat oven to 350°.
2. Put chopped tomatoes into boiling water and let sit.
3. Combine chicken and wine in baking dish and sprinkle with Italian seasoning.
4. Bake for 25–30 minutes or until juices run clear from chicken.
5. Remove and shred chicken.
6. Drain tomatoes; set aside juice.
7. Pour juices into sauté pan and sauté chicken and garlic over low heat for 5 minutes. Remove pan from heat.
8. Boil penne according to directions on package.
9. Spray small saucepan with cooking spray. Add flour and milk. Bring to a boil, stirring constantly. Lower heat and cook until thick.
10. Drain pasta and transfer to a pasta bowl.
11. Add chicken, chopped tomatoes, and sauce to pasta and mix well.

Great low-fat entrée with lots of calcium.

Nutrient Analysis (per serving): 421 calories, 18% calories from fat, 8% from saturated fat, iron 3 mg, vitamin C 2 mg, vitamin A 43 µg, calcium 271 mg, fiber 2 g.

Food Guide Pyramid: 2 ounces grain; ½ ounce meat; ¾ cups milk.

Recipe submitted by Christina Furtado while attending Region District #17, Higganum, CT.

Pizza à la Salad

Servings: 8
Oven temperature: 425°
Cooking time: 20 minutes

Amount	Measure	Ingredient
Pizza Dough:		
½	package	yeast
1¹/₃	cups	lukewarm water
1	tablespoon	sugar
4	cups	flour
2	teaspoons	vegetable shortening, melted
1	teaspoon	salt
Salad:		
½	bunch	romaine leaves, torn into pieces
½	head	iceberg lettuce
	desired amounts of:	cherry tomatoes, halves
		carrots, diced
		black olives, sliced
		red onion, chopped
		garlic powder

Instructions:

1. Mix yeast with warm water and sugar. Let sit about 5 minutes until yeast dissolves and becomes bubbly.
2. Mix flour, shortening, and salt. Add yeast mixture.
3. Knead about 10 minutes; add more flour if dough is too sticky.
4. Let dough rise in oiled bowl, covered with kitchen towel or plastic wrap, for about 1 hour, until double in size. Punch dough down and let sit about 15 minutes.
5. Roll dough on floured surface and transfer to pizza pan.
6. Bake in 425° oven for 20 minutes until golden brown.

7. Mix romaine and iceberg lettuce.
8. Put on top of pizza crust and top with vegetables.

A really healthy pizza. If you don't have enough time, use a prepared pizza crust.

Nutrient Analysis (per serving): 287 calories, 10% calories from fat, 1% from saturated fat, iron 4 mg, vitamin C 15 mg, vitamin A 1,599 µg, calcium 33 mg, fiber 4 g.

Food Guide Pyramid: 3 ounces grain; 2 cups vegetable; ½ teaspoon fats, oils, and sweets.

Recipe for dough submitted by Ginny Fatek and Mary Brundage while attending Bennie Dover Jackson Middle School, New London, CT.

Recipe for salad submitted by Roberto Fontan while attending Central High School, Bridgeport, CT.

Pizza Sauce

Servings: approx. 20
Cooking time: 10 minutes

Amount	Measure	Ingredient
2	tablespoons	oil
2	medium	onions, chopped
4	medium	garlic cloves, minced
1	28-ounce can	whole tomatoes
1	8-ounce can	tomato sauce
1	6-ounce can	tomato paste
2	teaspoons	oregano
2	teaspoons	basil
1½	tablespoons	chili powder
2	teaspoons	sugar
		salt and pepper to taste

Instructions:

1. Heat oil in medium saucepan. Add chopped onions and garlic and sauté until lightly browned.
2. Add tomatoes (crushing them if desired), tomato sauce, and tomato paste.
3. Bring to a boil and simmer for 5 minutes, stirring frequently.
4. Add seasonings and simmer about 10 minutes.

Enough sauce for two pizzas.
Try the pizza dough from Pizza à la Salad.

Nutrient Analysis (per serving): 42 calories, 31% calories from fat, 4% from saturated fat, iron 1 mg, vitamin C 9 mg, vitamin A 193 µg, calcium 24 mg, fiber 1 g.

Food Guide Pyramid: 1 cup vegetable.

Recipe submitted by Ginny Fatek and Mary Brundage while attending Bennie Dover Jackson Middle School, New London, CT.

Salmon Cakes

Servings: 4
Cooking time: 8 minutes

Amount	Measure	Ingredient
1	can	14 ¾-ounces red or pink salmon, drained and flaked
1	each	green onion, sliced
¼	cup	breadcrumbs
1	each	egg, beaten
¼	teaspoon	salt
¼	teaspoon	black pepper
1	tablespoon	mayonnaise
1	tablespoon	canola oil
4		sandwich buns, whole wheat

Instructions:

1. In a medium bowl, combine salmon, green onion, 2 tablespoons breadcrumbs, egg, salt, pepper, and mayonnaise. Lightly mix with fork.
2. Shape mixture into four 3-inch round patties and roll in remaining bread crumbs.
3. Heat oil in skillet. Add salmon cakes, and cook about 5 minutes per side over medium heat until golden brown.
4. Serve on whole wheat buns.

Salmon is a superfood—a great source of omega-fatty acids.

Nutrient Analysis (per serving): 448 calories, 41% calories from fat, 8% from saturated fat, iron 3 mg, vitamin C 1 mg, vitamin A 59 µg, calcium 260 mg, fiber 5 g.

Food Guide Pyramid: 2½ ounces grain; 2½ ounces meat; 1¼ teaspoons fats, oils, and sweets.

Sausage and Spinach Quiche

Servings: 8
Oven temperature: 350°–400°
Cooking time: 55 minutes

Amount	Measure	Ingredient
1	9-inch	pie crust
1	teaspoon	vegetable oil
1	pound	sweet Italian sausage, cut into chunks
¾	cup	onion, chopped
1	clove	garlic, minced
2	cups	mushrooms, sliced
1	10-oz pkg.	frozen spinach, thawed and chopped
3	medium	eggs
2	cups	mozzarella cheese, shredded
1	cup	provolone cheese, shredded
¾	cup	ricotta cheese
2	tablespoons	flour
1/8	teaspoon	pepper

Instructions:

1. Preheat oven to 400°.
2. Prick bottom of pie shell and bake for 5 minutes.
3. Remove from oven and reduce heat to 350°.
4. Heat oil in skillet and add sausage. Stir frequently for approximately 10 minutes until thoroughly cooked.
5. Add onion and garlic and cook for 5 minutes.
6. Add spinach and cook for 1 minute.
7. Remove and cool.
8. In medium bowl, beat eggs and stir in three cheeses, flour, and pepper.

continued on next page

9. Add egg mixture to sausage mixture and pour into partially cooked shell.
10. Bake for 30 minutes, or until knife inserted in center comes out clean.

Eggs are a superfood—a great source of vitamin A and calcium.

Nutrient Analysis (per serving): 499 calories, 65% calories from fat, 29% from saturated fat, iron 3 mg, vitamin C 11 mg, vitamin A 995 µg, calcium 389 mg, fiber 2 g.

Food Guide Pyramid: 1 ounce grain; 1 cup vegetable; 1 ounce meat; 1½ teaspoons fats, oils, and sweets.

Recipe submitted by Kevin Patterson while attending Waterford High School, Waterford, CT.

Taco Salad

Servings: 4
Oven temperature: 350°
Cooking time: 25 minutes

Amount	Measure	Ingredient
4	6-inch or 8-inch	corn tortillas
¾	pound	lean ground beef or turkey
1	medium	onion, chopped
1	medium	garlic clove, minced
1	8-ounce can	tomato sauce
1	teaspoon	vinegar
½	teaspoon	ground cumin
¼	teaspoon	crushed red pepper
4	cups	shredded lettuce
½	cup	green or red pepper, chopped
12	each	cherry tomatoes, halved
¼	cup	cheddar cheese, shredded

Instructions:

1. Wrap tortillas in foil and warm in a 350° oven for 10 minutes.
2. Spray four 10-ounce custard cups with nonstick cooking spray.
3. Carefully press 1 tortilla into each cup.
4. Bake in a 350° oven for 15 minutes or until crisp. Cool and remove from custard cups.
5. In large skillet, cook meat, onion, and garlic until meat is no longer pink and onion is tender.
6. Drain fat and stir in tomato sauce, vinegar, cumin, and crushed red pepper.
7. Bring mixture to a boil, reduce heat, and simmer for 10 minutes.
8. Place each tortilla on a plate. Add lettuce, peppers, and tomatoes.
9. Divide beef mixture evenly on top of salad. Top with cheese.

continued on next page

Good source of vitamins, minerals, and fiber.

Nutrient Analysis (per serving): 358 calories, 41% calories from fat, 16% from saturated fat, iron 3 mg, vitamin C 51 mg, vitamin A 975 µg, calcium 111 mg, fiber 5 g.

Food Guide Pyramid: 1 ounce grain; 3 cups vegetable; 1 ounce meat; ½ teaspoon fats, oils, and sweets.

Recipe submitted by Suzanne Johnston while attending Waterford High School, Waterford, CT, and Mike Pugliese while attending Region District #5, Bethany, CT.

Three Cheese Macaroni

Servings: 6
Oven temperature: 350°
Cooking time: 30 minutes

Amount	Measure	Ingredient
3	cups	macaroni (cooked and drained)
1	11-ounce can	condensed cheddar cheese soup
1	cup	reduced-fat (2%) milk
½	teaspoon	ground mustard
¼	teaspoon	seasoned salt
½	cup	Swiss cheese, shredded
½	cup	cheddar cheese, shredded
½	cup	grated parmesan cheese
1	2.8-ounce can	french-fried onions

Instructions:

1. Preheat oven to 350°.
2. Combine cooked macaroni, soup, milk, ground mustard, salt, ¼ cup of each cheese, and ½ can of onions in casserole dish.
3. Bake covered for 25 minutes.
4. Top with remaining cheeses and onions.
5. Bake uncovered for an additional 5 minutes.

More than one-third of your daily calcium in a serving of this tasty dish.

Nutrient Analysis (per serving): 333 calories, 41% calories from fat, 18% from saturated fat, iron 1 mg, vitamin C 0 mg, vitamin A 208 µg, calcium 377 mg, fiber 1 g.

continued on next page

Food Guide Pyramid: 1 ounce grain; 1 cup milk; ½ teaspoon fats, oils, and sweets.

Recipe submitted by Pat Adorno, teacher, Klingberg Family Center, Inc., New Britain, CT.

SNACKS

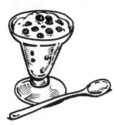

Applesauce

Servings: 4
Cooking time: 5–10 minutes

Amount	Measure	Ingredient
4	medium	apples
½	cup	water
¼	cup	raisins
¼	cup	sugar
¼	teaspoon	cinnamon
¼	cup	walnuts, chopped
4	scoops	vanilla ice cream or frozen yogurt (optional)

Instructions:

1. Cut apples into quarters and slice into pieces, leaving peel on apple.
2. Place apples and water in medium saucepan.
3. Bring to a boil over medium heat.
4. Reduce heat and add raisins. Simmer for 5–10 minutes, stirring occasionally.
5. Stir in sugar, cinnamon, and chopped walnuts. Heat to boil.
6. Serve in individual bowls.

continued on next page

Additional serving ideas:

Serve over scoop of ice cream or frozen yogurt. Use as topping for pancakes, quick breads, or bagels.

Good source of fiber. Nuts are one of those superfoods.

Nutrient Analysis (per serving): 189 calories, 22% calories from fat, 2% from saturated fat, iron 1 mg, vitamin C 7 mg, vitamin A 21 µg, calcium 22 mg, fiber 4 g.

Food Guide Pyramid: 1 cup fruit; 3½ teaspoons fats, oils, and sweets.

Recipe submitted by Marilyn Schwab, teacher, Fair Haven Middle School, New Haven, CT.

Blueberry Parfait

Servings: 1

Amount	Measure	Ingredient
½	cup	blueberries, fresh or frozen (thawed)
4	tablespoons	fat-free lemon yogurt
2	2½-inch squares	graham crackers, crumbled

Instructions:

1. Layer ¼ cup blueberries, 2 tablespoons yogurt, and 1 crumbled graham cracker in parfait glass.
2. Repeat layers.

Great dessert or snack. Get lots of antioxidants, and it's low-fat too.

Nutrient Analysis (per serving): 156 calories, 10% calories from fat, 2% from saturated fat, iron 1 mg, vitamin C 10 mg, vitamin A 23 µg, calcium 117 mg, fiber 2 g.

Food Guide Pyramid: ½ serving grain; 1 cup fruit; ½ cup milk; 2 teaspoons fats, oils, and sweets.

Recipe submitted by Rebecca Shwartz while attending Region District #5, Bethany, CT.

Colleen's Granola

Servings: 8

Amount	Measure	Ingredient
3	cups	rolled oats
¼	cup	Grape Nuts cereal or other nugget cereal
½	cup	walnuts, chopped or other nuts
1/3	cup	brown sugar
¼	cup	honey
1	teaspoon	cinnamon
1	teaspoon	vanilla
1/3	cup	canola oil
1	cup	raisins

Instructions:

1. Preheat oven to 350°. Spray a 9-inch by 13-inch pan with cooking spray.
2. Combine all ingredients except raisins in a large mixing bowl. Transfer to prepared pan. Bake for 20 minutes, stirring occasionally.
3. Remove from oven and immediately add raisins.
4. Transfer to large cookie sheet. Spread out evenly to cool.
5. Store in an airtight container.

Contains two superfoods: oats and nuts.

Nutrient Analysis (per serving): 342 calories, 20% calories from fat, 6% from saturated fat, iron 3 mg, vitamin C 0 mg, vitamin A 16 µg, calcium 13 mg, fiber 4 g.

Food Guide Pyramid: 1½ servings grain; 1 cup fruit; 2 teaspoons fats, oils, and sweets.

Recipe by Colleen Thompson, MS, RD.

Hummus

Servings: 10

Amount	Measure	Ingredient
½	medium	garlic cloves
½	teaspoon	salt
¼	teaspoon	pepper
1/8	teaspoon	paprika
1/8	teaspoon	cayenne pepper
2	cups	chickpeas (garbanzo beans), drained and liquid reserved
1	small bunch	fresh parsley (save approx. ½ for garnishing)

Instructions:

1. Combine all ingredients in food processor except for reserved liquid and parsley garnish.
2. Run food processor until mixture's consistency is smooth.
3. Adjust seasonings to taste, and add reserved liquid to make desired consistency.
4. Serve garnished with fresh parsley.

Try serving this with pita chips, a spread, or a dip. Great instead of mayo on a sandwich.

Nutrient Analysis (per serving): 50 calories, 18% calories from fat, 0% from saturated fat, iron 1 mg, vitamin C 4 mg, vitamin A 55 µg, calcium 21 mg, fiber 3 g.

Food Guide Pyramid: Dip is not a significant source of any food group.

Recipe submitted by Marjorie Wheeler, teacher, Westbrook High School, Westbrook, CT.

Mudd Dip

Servings: 6

Amount	Measure	Ingredient
1	15½-ounce can	kidney beans or cannellini beans
1	tablespoon	vinegar
1	teaspoon	chili powder
1/8	teaspoon	cumin
2	teaspoons	onion, minced
2	teaspoons	parsley

Instructions:

1. Drain kidney beans or cannellini beans and reserve liquid.
2. Place beans, vinegar, chili powder, and cumin in blender. Blend until smooth, adding reserved liquid as needed.
3. Stir in onion and parsley and chill thoroughly.

The dip is good served with whole-wheat crackers or crisp vegetable sticks.

Beans are a great fiber source and superfood.

Nutrient Analysis (per serving): 68 calories, 4% calories from fat, 0% from saturated fat, iron 1 mg, vitamin C 2 mg, vitamin A 51 µg, calcium 22 mg, fiber 5 g.

Food Guide Pyramid: Dip is not a significant source of any food group.

Recipe submitted by Carolyn Brennan, Providers Nutrition Network, Plainville, CT.

Peanut Butter Apple Wedges

Servings: 1

Amount	Measure	Ingredient
1	8-inch	flour tortilla
2	tablespoons	peanut butter
2	tablespoons	apples, peeled, cored, and chopped*

*Bananas may be substituted for apples.

Instructions:

1. Spread peanut butter onto tortilla.
2. Sprinkle apples on peanut butter.
3. Fold tortillas and cut into wedges.

An easy after-school snack.

Nutrient Analysis (per serving): 305 calories, 54% calories from fat, 12% from saturated fat, iron 1 mg, vitamin C 1 mg, vitamin A 2 µg, calcium 13 mg, fiber 4 g.

Food Guide Pyramid: ½ ounce grain; ½ ounce meat; 1 teaspoon fats, oils, and sweets.

Recipe submitted by Tiffany Chen while attending Region District #5, Bethany, CT.

Spinach Dip for Veggies

Servings: 6

Amount	Measure	Ingredient
1	cup	low-fat cottage cheese
1	cup	fat-free plain yogurt
2	cups	fresh spinach, washed, dried, and chopped
3	medium	garlic cloves, minced
1/8	teaspoon	black pepper, ground
1	pinch	nutmeg
		assorted vegetables of choice

Instructions:

1. Mix all ingredients until well combined.
2. Serve with vegetables.

Serve as a dip or use as a spread. Tastes super and has a super dairy food: yogurt.

Nutrient Analysis (per serving): 33 calories, 8% calories from fat, 5% from saturated fat, iron 0 mg, vitamin C 2 mg, vitamin A 137 µg, calcium 57 mg, fiber 0 g.

Food Guide Pyramid: Dip is not a significant source of any food group.

Recipe submitted by Cindy Connor, RD, Millbrook, NY.

Sweet and Sour Fruit Dressing

Servings: 12

Amount	Measure	Ingredient
1	cup	vanilla fat-free yogurt
1	tablespoon	honey
6–7	medium	strawberries
¼	cup	raisins or dried cranberries
½	cup	kiwi fruit

Instructions:

1. Put all ingredients into blender or food processor and blend until smooth.
2. Refrigerate until ready to serve.

Kiwi is a super fruit. Serve over the fruits of your choice, or use as a dip for fruit.

Nutrient Analysis (per serving): 37 calories, 3% calories from fat, 1% from saturated fat, iron 0 mg, vitamin C 11 mg, vitamin A 5 µg, calcium 37 mg, fiber 1 g.

Food Guide Pyramid: 1 teaspoon fats, oils, and sweets.

Recipe submitted by Elicia Masztal while attending Region District #17, Higganum, CT.

Whole-Wheat Pretzels

Servings: 16
Oven temperature: 400°
Cooking time: 15 minutes

Amount	Measure	Ingredient
1	cup	lukewarm water
1½	teaspoon	yeast
½	cup	sugar
1	teaspoon	salt
2	tablespoons	margarine, softened
½	medium	egg
1¼–3	cups	all-purpose flour
1	cup	whole-wheat flour
½	large	egg yolk
1	tablespoon	water
½	tablespoon	coarse salt

Instructions:

1. Mix yeast with warm water. Let sit about 5 minutes until yeast dissolves and becomes bubbly.
2. Add sugar, salt, margarine, egg, ½ cup all-purpose flour, and 1 cup whole-wheat flour.
3. Stir until smooth. Add enough flour to make a stiff dough.
4. Turn onto a lightly floured surface and divide into 16 pieces.
5. Roll each piece into a 20-inch long rope and shape into a pretzel by bringing the ends to the center.
6. Place on lightly greased cookie sheet and refrigerate for at least 2 hours but not more than 24 hours.
7. Preheat oven to 400°.
8. Blend yolk and 1 tablespoon of water, brush onto pretzels, and top with coarse salt.
9. Bake at 400° for 15 minutes.

Whole-grain and a great low-fat snack.

Nutrient Analysis (per serving): 138 calories, 13% calories from fat, 3% from saturated fat, iron 1 mg, vitamin C 0 mg, vitamin A 22 µg, calcium 9 mg, fiber 1 g.

Food Guide Pyramid: 1½ ounces grain; 1½ teaspoons fats, oils, and sweets.

Recipe submitted by Cindy VanFleet, teacher, Platt High School, Meriden, CT.

Apple Walnut Crisp

Servings: 8
Oven temperature: 375°
Cooking time: 40 minutes

Amount	Measure	Ingredient
½	cup	all-purpose flour
¾	cup	old-fashioned rolled oats
½	cup	light brown sugar, packed
½	teaspoon	salt
4	tablespoons	butter, softened
¼	cup	walnuts, chopped
3	pounds	apples, McIntosh, peeled and sliced, or your choice of apple
2	tablespoons	lemon juice
1	tablespoon	Sugar

Instructions:

1. Preheat oven to 375°.
2. In a bowl, mix together first four ingredients for topping. Add butter and blend until mixture looks like coarse meal. This may be done in a food processor. Stir in walnuts.
3. In large bowl, toss apples, lemon juice, and sugar.
4. Spray a 2-quart dish with cooking spray. Spread apple mixture into prepared pan. Crumble topping over apple.
5. Place in preheated oven for about 30 minutes, or until apples are tender. Remove from oven and let sit for 10 minutes.

Easy to prepare and a great source of fiber. Has 2 superfoods: oats and nuts.

Nutrient Analysis (per serving): 283 calories, 28% calories from fat, 12% calories from saturated fat, iron 2 mg, vitamin C 2 mg, vitamin A 62 µg, calcium 35 mg, fiber 6 g.

Food Guide Pyramid: ½ ounce grain; 1¼ cups fruit; 2 teaspoons fats, oils, and sweets.

DESSERTS

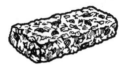

Energy Bars

Servings: 30
Oven temperature: 350°
Cooking time: 15 minutes

Amount	Measure	Ingredient
1½	cup	quick oats
1	cup	brown rice cereal
¼	cup	sesame seeds
3	cups	mixture of dried fruit (apricots, raisins, cranberries, etc.)
½	cup	dry milk
½	cup	toasted wheat germ
1	cup	light corn syrup
½	cup	sugar
½	cup	natural peanut butter
1½	teaspoon	vanilla extract
½	teaspoon	cinnamon

Instructions:

1. Preheat oven to 350°.
2. Spread oats, rice cereal, and sesame seeds on 8-inch by 13-inch jelly roll pan. Bake, stirring occasionally until oats are toasted.
3. Chop fruit so it is a similar size. Do not need to chop raisins and cranberries. Put in large bowl.
4. Add dry milk and wheat germ to fruit. Toss to mix.

5. Stir hot oatmeal mixture into fruit.
6. Spray jelly roll pan with cooking spray.
7. In a heavy saucepan, combine corn syrup and sugar. Bring to a boil over medium heat. Reduce heat to low and stir in peanut butter, vanilla, and cinnamon.
8. Quickly pour syrup mixture over oatmeal and mix well.
9. Spread warm mixture onto prepared pan. Spread evenly, pressing into a thin layer.
10. Chill until firm. Cut into bars. Can be stored up to month in the refrigerator.

A tasty energy treat. Oats is a superfood.

Nutrient analysis (per serving): 148 calories, 4% calories from fat, 2% calories from saturated fat, iron 1 mg, vitamin C 1 mg, vitamin A 24 µg, calcium 35 mg, fiber 3 g.

Food Guide Pyramid: ¼ ounce grain; ¾ cup fruit; 1 teaspoons fats, oils, and sweets.

Recipe by University of New Haven Nutrition and Dietetics.

Oatmeal Apple Cookies

Servings: 18 (2 cookies each)
Oven temperature: 375°
Cooking time: 10–12 minutes

Amount	Measure	Ingredient
1	cup	flour
1	teaspoon	baking powder
¼	teaspoon	salt
1/8	teaspoon	cinnamon
1	cup	dark brown sugar, firmly packed
½	cup	butter or margarine
1	large	egg
½	teaspoon	vanilla
1½	cup	rolled oats
½		tart apple, peeled and finely chopped

Instructions:

1. In a small bowl, combine flour, baking powder, salt, and cinnamon.
2. In a large bowl, combine brown sugar and butter; beat until light and fluffy.
3. Beat in egg and vanilla.
4. Add flour mixture and rolled oats separately to creamed mixture, blending well after each addition.
5. Stir in apples.
6. Drop by rounded teaspoonful onto ungreased cookie sheets. Makes 36 cookies.
7. Bake 10–12 minutes, or until lightly browned.

Oats is a superfood.

Nutrient analysis (per serving): 136 calories, 9% calories from fat, 17% calories from saturated fat, iron 1 mg, vitamin C 0 mg, vitamin A 479 µg, calcium 2 mg, fiber 1 g.

Food Guide Pyramid: ½ ounce grain; 2 teaspoons fats, oils, and sweets.

Recipe submitted by Tina Twiggs, teacher, Sheehan High School, Wallingford, CT.

Raspberry Pie

Servings: 8
Preparation time: 20 minutes

Amount	Measure	Ingredient
1	3-ounce package	raspberry gelatin
2/3	cup	hot water
2	cups	ice cubes
1	9-inch	graham cracker crust
1	8-ounce container	frozen low-fat whipped topping, thawed
1½	cups	raspberries
		chopped nuts (optional)

Instructions:

1. Dissolve gelatin in hot water.
2. Add about 2 cups of ice cubes to thicken quickly.
3. Pour gelatin into graham cracker pie crust.
4. Spread whipped topping evenly over gelatin.
5. Spoon raspberries over whipped topping.
6. Top with chopped nuts (optional).
7. Chill in refrigerator until set and ready to serve.

Nutrient Analysis (per serving): 243 calories, 15% calories from fat, 29% calories from saturated fat, iron 1 mg, vitamin C 8 mg, vitamin A 9 μg, calcium 33 mg, fiber 2 g.

Food Guide Pyramid: ¼ cup fruit; 1 ounce meat; 4 teaspoons fats, oils, and sweets.

Recipe submitted by Megan Cebulski, student, Hillcrest Middle School, Trumbull, CT.

Strawberry Trifle

Servings: 10

Amount	Measure	Ingredient
1	package	sugar-free vanilla instant pudding
1	cup	low-fat milk
1	8-ounce container	light whipped topping, thawed
1	10-inch	angel food cake, cut into bite-sized pieces
2	pints	fresh strawberries, hulled and sliced (could substitute frozen)

Instructions:

1. In large bowl, mix pudding and milk until thickened.
2. Fold in whipped topping.
3. In large glass serving bowl, layer ½ cake pieces, 1/3 of strawberries, and ½ pudding mixture. Repeat layers, finishing with strawberries.
4. Cover and refrigerate at least 2 hours.

Strawberries are a super fruit. Really easy and tastes great.

Nutrient Analysis (per serving): 178 calories, 6% calories from fat, 14% calories from saturated fat, iron 0 mg, vitamin C 34 mg, vitamin A 23 µg, calcium 108 mg, fiber 2 g.

Food Guide Pyramid: 1/3 cup fruit; 2½ teaspoons fats, oils, and sweets

Recipe submitted by Tina Dugdale, MS, RN, RD.

Sugar and Spice Pecans

Servings: 10
Oven temperature: 300°
Cooking time: 30 minutes

Amount	Measure	Ingredient
1	large	egg white
1	tablespoon	water
2½	cup	whole pecans
½	cup	sugar
1	teaspoon	cinnamon

Instructions:

1. Beat egg white with fork until frothy. Add water and beat.
2. Mix sugar and cinnamon and add to egg white mixture. Blend well with fork.
3. Pour egg mixture on pecans and mix well, coating all pecans.
4. Spread on cookie sheet sprayed with cooking spray. Bake for 15 minutes.
5. Turn pecans with spatula and bake an additional 15 minutes.
6. Spread on foil to cool.

Great tasting. Put a few on a salad to add an extra crunch.

Nutrient Analysis (per serving): 229 calories, 30% calories from fat, 8% calories from saturated fat, iron 1 mg, vitamin C 0 mg, vitamin A 5 µg, calcium 19 mg, fiber 3 g.

Food Guide Pyramid: 1/3 ounce meat; 4 teaspoons fats, oils, and sweets.

Recipe by Ann O'Brien, RD.

Sweet Potato Pudding

Servings: 10
Oven temperature: 350°
Cooking time: 1–1½ hours

Amount	Measure	Ingredient
1 ¼	pounds	sweet potato, grated
½	cup	flour
¼	cup	yellow cornmeal
2	tablespoons	raisins
½	teaspoon	baking powder
1	cup	fat-free evaporated milk
2	cups	reduced-fat coconut milk
¾	cup	brown sugar
1	teaspoon	vanilla
¼	teaspoon	nutmeg
¼	teaspoon	salt
1	ounce	butter, melted

Instructions:

1. Preheat oven to 350°. Grease a 9-inch by 13-inch pan.
2. Mix grated sweet potatoes with flour, cornmeal, raisins, and baking powder.
3. In another bowl, combine evaporated milk, coconut milk, sugar, vanilla, nutmeg, salt, and melted butter. Mix well.
4. Pour milk mixture into potato mixture and mix until smooth.
5. Pour into prepared pan and let rest for 30 minutes. Bake in oven for 1 to 1½ hours, until center is set.
6. Serve hot or cold.

Sweet potatoes are one of those superfoods. Great dessert.

continued on next page

Nutrient Analysis (per serving): 179 calories, 8% calories from fat, 19% calories from saturated fat, iron 1 mg, vitamin C 1 mg, vitamin A 182 µg, calcium 78 mg, fiber 1 g.

Food Guide Pyramid: ½ ounce grain; ¾ cup vegetable; ¼ cup milk; 2 teaspoons fats, oils, and sweets.

Recipe by Lellieth Keize.

Appendix A
Dietary Reference Intakes (DRIs) : Recommended Intakes of Select Vitamins, Minerals, and Macronutrients for Teens*

	Males		Females		
	9–13	14–18	9–13	14–18	
Vit A	600	900	600	700	µg
Vit C	45	75	45	65	mg
Vit D	5	5	5	5	µg
Folic Acid	300	400	300	400	µg
Niacin	12	16	12	14	mg
Thiamin	0.9	1.2	0.9	1	mg
Riboflavin	0.9	1.3	0.9	1	mg
B-6	1	1.3	1	1.2	mg
B-12	1.8	2.4	1.8	2.4	µg
Vit E	11	15	11	15	mg
Calcium	1300	1300	1300	1300	mg
Sodium	1.5	1.5	1.5	1.5	g
Iron	8	11	8	15	mg
Zinc	8	11	8	9	mg
Macronutrients					
Carbohydrate	130	130	130	130	g
Protein	34	52	34	46	g
Fat	ND†	ND	ND	ND	g
Fiber	31	38	26	26	g

* DRIs are developed by National Academy of Sciences. Institute of Medicine. Food and Nutrition Board. The complete listing may be found at http://fnic.nal.usda.gov/nal_display/index.php?info_center=4&tax_level=3&tax_subject=256&topic_id=1342&level3_id=5140

† ND = Not determinable due to lack of data about adverse effects in this age group and concern with regard to lack of ability to handle excess amounts. Source of intake should be from food only, to prevent high levels of intake.

Estimated Calories Needed by Gender, Age, and Activity Level[a]

	Males		Females	
	9–13	14–18	9–13	14–18
Sedentary[b]	1800	2200	1600	1800
Moderately Active[c]	1800–2200[e]	2400–2800	1600–2000	2000
Active[d]	2000–2600	2800–3200	2200	2400

a These levels are based on Estimated Energy Requirements (EER) from the Institute of Medicine (IOM) Dietary Reference Intakes macronutrients report, 2002, calculated by gender,
age, and activity level for reference-sized individuals. Reference size, as determined by IOM,
is based on median height and weight for ages up to 18 years and median height and weight
for that height to give a Body Mass Index (BMI) of 21.5 for adult females and 22.5 for adult
males.

b A lifestyle that includes only the light physical activity associated with typical day-to-day life.

c A lifestyle that includes physical activity equivalent to walking about 1.5 to 3 miles per day
at 3 to 4 miles per hour, in addition to the light physical activity associated with typical day-
to-day life.

d A lifestyle that includes physical activity equivalent to walking more than 3 miles per day at
3 to 4 miles per hour, in addition to the light physical activity associated with typical day-to-
day life.

e The calorie ranges shown are to accommodate needs of different ages within the group. For
children and adolescents, more calories are needed at older ages. For adults, fewer calories
are needed at older ages.

Note: The complete table may be found at
www.health.gov/dietaryguidelines/dga2005/toolkit/healthfacts/weight.htm.

Appendix B
Exercise Calorie Expenditures from Nutribase (30 minutes)

Activity	90 lbs.	100 lbs.	110 lbs.	120 lbs.	130 lbs.	140 lbs.	150 lbs.
Aerobic dancing (low-impact)	104	115	127	138	149	161	172
Aerobics step 4" step (beginner)	131	145	160	174	189	203	218
Aerobics, slide training (basic)	135	150	165	180	195	210	225
Backpacking with 10 lb. load	162	180	198	216	234	252	270
Backpacking with 20 lb. load	180	200	220	240	260	280	300
Backpacking with 30 lb. load	211	235	259	282	306	329	352
Badminton	135	150	165	180	195	210	225
Basketball (game)	198	220	242	264	286	308	330
Basketball (leisurely, nongame)	117	130	143	156	169	182	195
Bicycling, 10 mph (6 min/mile)	112	125	138	150	162	175	188
Bicycling, 13 mph (4.6 min/mile)	180	200	220	240	260	280	300
Billiards	41	45	49	54	58	63	68
Bowling	50	55	60	66	72	77	82

160 lbs.	170 lbs.	180 lbs.	190 lbs.	200 lbs.	220 lbs.	240 lbs.	260 lbs.	280 lbs.	300 lbs.
184	195	207	218	230	253	276	299	322	345
232	247	261	276	290	319	348	377	406	435
240	255	270	285	300	330	360	390	420	450
288	306	324	342	360	396	432	468	504	540
320	340	360	380	400	440	480	520	560	600
376	399	423	446	470	517	564	611	658	705
240	255	270	285	300	330	360	390	420	450
352	374	396	418	440	484	528	572	616	660
208	221	234	247	260	286	312	338	364	390
200	213	225	237	250	275	300	325	350	375
320	340	360	380	400	440	480	520	560	600
72	76	81	85	90	99	108	117	126	135
88	94	99	105	110	121	132	143	154	165

Appendix B
Exercise Calorie Expenditures from Nutribase (30 minutes)

Activity	90 lbs.	100 lbs.	110 lbs.	120 lbs.	130 lbs.	140 lbs.	150 lbs.
Canoeing, 2.5 mph	63	70	77	84	91	98	105
Canoeing, 4.0 mph	122	135	149	162	175	189	202
Croquet	54	60	66	72	78	84	90
Cross country snow skiing, intense	297	330	363	396	429	462	495
Cross country snow skiing, leisurely	140	155	171	186	202	217	232
Cross country snow skiing, moderate	198	220	242	264	286	308	330
Dancing (noncontact)	90	100	110	120	130	140	150
Dancing (slow)	50	55	60	66	72	77	82
Gardening, moderate	81	90	99	108	117	126	135
Golfing (walking, w/o cart)	90	100	110	120	130	140	150
Golfing (with a cart)	63	70	77	84	91	98	105
Handball	207	230	253	276	299	322	345

160 lbs.	170 lbs.	180 lbs.	190 lbs.	200 lbs.	220 lbs.	240 lbs.	260 lbs.	280 lbs.	300 lbs.
112	119	126	133	140	154	168	182	196	210
216	230	243	257	270	297	324	351	378	405
96	102	108	114	120	132	144	156	168	180
528	561	594	627	660	726	792	858	924	990
248	263	279	294	310	341	372	403	434	465
352	374	396	418	440	484	528	572	616	660
160	170	180	190	200	220	240	260	280	300
88	94	99	105	110	121	132	143	154	165
144	153	162	171	180	198	216	234	252	270
160	170	180	190	200	220	240	260	280	300
112	119	126	133	140	154	168	182	196	210
368	391	414	437	460	506	552	598	644	690

Appendix B
Exercise Calorie Expenditures from Nutribase (30 minutes)

Activity	90 lbs.	100 lbs.	110 lbs.	120 lbs.	130 lbs.	140 lbs.	150 lbs.
Hiking with a 10 lb. load	162	180	198	216	234	252	270
Hiking with a 20 lb. load	180	200	220	240	260	280	300
Hiking with a 30 lb. load	211	235	259	282	306	329	352
Hiking, no load	140	155	171	186	202	217	232
Housework	81	90	99	108	117	126	135
Ironing	45	50	55	60	65	70	75
Jogging, 5 mph (12 min/mile)	167	185	203	222	240	259	278
Jogging, 6 mph (10 min/mile)	207	230	253	276	299	322	345
Mopping	77	85	94	102	111	119	128
Mowing	122	135	149	162	175	189	202
Ping Pong	81	90	99	108	117	126	135
Raking	68	75	82	90	98	105	112
Racquetball	185	205	225	246	266	287	308
Rowing (leisurely)	68	75	82	90	98	105	112
Rowing machine	162	180	198	216	234	252	270

160 lbs.	170 lbs.	180 lbs.	190 lbs.	200 lbs.	220 lbs.	240 lbs.	260 lbs.	280 lbs.	300 lbs.
288	306	324	342	360	396	432	468	504	540
320	340	360	380	400	440	480	520	560	600
376	399	423	446	470	517	564	611	658	705
248	263	279	294	310	341	372	403	434	465
144	153	162	171	180	198	216	234	252	270
80	85	90	95	100	110	120	130	140	150
296	315	333	352	370	407	444	481	518	555
368	391	414	437	460	506	552	598	644	690
136	144	153	162	170	187	204	221	238	255
216	230	243	257	270	297	324	351	378	405
144	153	162	171	180	198	216	234	252	270
120	128	135	142	150	165	180	195	210	225
328	349	369	389	410	451	492	533	574	615
120	128	135	142	150	165	180	195	210	225
288	306	324	342	360	396	432	468	504	540

Appendix B
Exercise Calorie Expenditures from Nutribase (30 minutes)

Activity	90 lbs.	100 lbs.	110 lbs.	120 lbs.	130 lbs.	140 lbs.	150 lbs.
Running, 08 mph (7.5 min/mile)	274	305	336	366	396	427	458
Running, 09 mph (6.7 min/mile)	297	330	363	396	429	462	495
Running, 10 mph (6 min/mile)	315	350	385	420	455	490	525
Scrubbing the floor	126	140	154	168	182	196	210
Scuba diving	171	190	209	228	247	266	285
Shopping for groceries	54	60	66	72	78	84	90
Skipping rope	257	285	313	342	370	399	428
Snow shoveling	176	195	215	234	253	273	292
Snow skiing, downhill	117	130	143	156	169	182	195
Soccer	176	195	215	234	253	273	292
Squash	185	205	225	246	266	287	308
Stair climber machine	144	160	176	192	208	224	240
Stair climbing	126	140	154	168	182	196	210
Swimming (25 yds/min)	108	120	132	144	156	168	180

160 lbs.	170 lbs.	180 lbs.	190 lbs.	200 lbs.	220 lbs.	240 lbs.	260 lbs.	280 lbs.	300 lbs.
488	518	549	579	610	671	732	793	854	915
528	561	594	627	660	726	792	858	924	990
560	595	630	665	700	770	840	910	980	1050
224	238	252	266	280	308	336	364	392	420
304	323	342	361	380	418	456	494	532	570
96	102	108	114	120	132	144	156	168	180
456	484	513	541	570	627	684	741	798	855
312	332	351	371	390	429	468	507	546	585
208	221	234	247	260	286	312	338	364	390
312	332	351	371	390	429	468	507	546	585
328	349	369	389	410	451	492	533	574	615
256	272	288	304	320	352	384	416	448	480
224	238	252	266	280	308	336	364	392	420
192	204	216	228	240	264	288	312	336	360

Appendix B
Exercise Calorie Expenditures from Nutribase (30 minutes)

Activity	90 lbs.	100 lbs.	110 lbs.	120 lbs.	130 lbs.	140 lbs.	150 lbs.
Swimming (50 yds/min)	202	225	248	270	292	315	338
Table Tennis	81	90	99	108	117	126	135
Tennis	144	160	176	192	208	224	240
Tennis (doubles)	99	110	121	132	143	154	165
Trimming hedges	94	105	115	126	136	147	158
Vacuuming	68	75	82	90	98	105	112
Volleyball (game)	108	120	132	144	156	168	180
Volleyball (leisurely)	63	70	77	84	91	98	105
Walking, 2 mph (30 min/mile)	54	60	66	72	78	84	90
Walking, 3 mph (20 min/mile)	72	80	88	96	104	112	120
Walking, 4 mph (15 min/mile)	90	100	110	120	130	140	150
Washing the car	68	75	82	90	98	105	112
Waterskiing	144	160	176	192	208	224	240
Waxing the car	90	100	110	120	130	140	150
Weeding	90	100	110	120	130	140	150

160 lbs.	170 lbs.	180 lbs.	190 lbs.	200 lbs.	220 lbs.	240 lbs.	260 lbs.	280 lbs.	300 lbs.
360	382	405	428	450	495	540	585	630	675
144	153	162	171	180	198	216	234	252	270
256	272	288	304	320	352	384	416	448	480
176	187	198	209	220	242	264	286	308	330
168	178	189	199	210	231	252	273	294	315
120	128	135	142	150	165	180	195	210	225
192	204	216	228	240	264	288	312	336	360
112	119	126	133	140	154	168	182	196	210
96	102	108	114	120	132	144	156	168	180
128	136	144	152	160	176	192	208	224	240
160	170	180	190	200	220	240	260	280	300
120	128	135	142	150	165	180	195	210	225
256	272	288	304	320	352	384	416	448	480
160	170	180	190	200	220	240	260	280	300
160	170	180	190	200	220	240	260	280	300

Appendix B
Exercise Calorie Expenditures from Nutribase (30 minutes)

Activity	90 lbs.	100 lbs.	110 lbs.	120 lbs.	130 lbs.	140 lbs.	150 lbs.
Weight training (40 sec. between sets)	230	255	280	306	332	357	382
Weight training (60 sec. between sets)	171	190	209	228	247	266	285
Weight training (90 sec. between sets)	112	125	138	150	162	175	188
Window cleaning	68	75	82	90	98	105	112

160 lbs.	170 lbs.	180 lbs.	190 lbs.	200 lbs.	220 lbs.	240 lbs.	260 lbs.	280 lbs.	300 lbs.
408	433	459	484	510	561	612	663	714	765
304	323	342	361	380	418	456	494	532	570
200	213	225	237	250	275	300	325	350	375
120	128	135	142	150	165	180	195	210	

References and Resources

Chapter 1: The Basics; Chapter 2: Find Your Fuel; Chapter 3: Vitamins and Minerals; Chapter 4: Let's Move

Centers for Disease Control and Prevention, "How Much Physical Activity Do You Need?" http://cdc.gov/physicalactivity/everyone/guidelines/index.html.

Henry J. Kaiser Family Foundation. www.kff.org.

Hoeger, Wener K., and Sharon A. Hoeger. 2009. *Lifetime Physical Fitness and Wellness: A Personalized Program,* 10th ed. Belmont, CA: Hoeger and Hoeger.

Mahan, L. Kathleen, and Sylvia Escott-Stump, eds. 2007. *Krause's Food, Nutrition & Diet Therapy,* 12th ed. St. Louis: W. B. Saunders Company.

Nemours. "Teens Health." http://kidshealth.org/teen/.

U.S. Department of Agriculture. "Food and Nutrition Information Center: Dietary Guidance." http://fnic.nal.usda.gov/nal_display/index.php?info_center=4&tax_level=3 &tax_subject=256&topic_id=1342&level3_id=5140.

U.S. Department of Agriculture. "Steps to a Healthier You." www.mypyramid.gov.

U.S. Department of Health and Human Services. "Dietary Guidelines for Americans," www.health.gov/dietaryguidelines/.

Chapter 5: Weight Management

Centers for Disease Control and Prevention, "Healthy Weight—It's Not a Diet, It's a Lifestyle!" www.cdc.gov/healthyweight/assessing/bmi/.

Chapter 6: Eating Disorders

Alpha Nutrition. "Eating Disorders." http://nutramed.com/eatingdisorders/index.htm.

American Dietetic Association. 2006. "Position of the American Dietetic Association: Nutrition Intervention in the Treatment of Anorexia Nervosa, Bulimia Nervosa, and Other Eating Disorders." *Journal of the American Dietetic Association* 106: 2073–2082.

Eating Disorder Foundation. www.eatingdisorderfoundation.org. 1 (303) 322-3373.

Hudson, J., E. Hiripi, H. Pope Jr., and R. Kessler. 2007. "The Prevalence and Correlates of Eating Disorders in the National Comorbidity Survey Replication." *Biological Psychiatry* 61(3): 348–358.

National Association of Anorexia Nervosa and Associated Disorders. www.anad.org. 1 (847) 831-3438.

National Eating Disorders Association. www.nationaleatingdisorders.org. 1 (206) 382-3587.

National Institute of Mental Health. 2007. "Study Tracks Prevalence of Eating Disorders." www.nimh.nih.gov/science-news/2007/study-tracks-prevalence-of-eating-disorders.shtml.

National Institute of Mental Health. 2008. *Eating Disorders.* www.nimh.nih.gov/health/publications/eating-disorders/complete-index.shtml.

Chapter 7: Vegetarianism

American Dietetic Association. 2009. "Position of the American Dietetic Association: Vegetarian Diets." *Journal of the American Dietetic Association* 109: 1266–1282.

Food and Agriculture Organization of the United Nations. 2006. "Livestock a Major Threat to Environment." www.fao.org/newsroom/en/news/2006/1000448/index.html.

Vegetarian Resource Group. www.vrg.org.

Veggie Table. "What Is a Vegetarian?" www.theveggietable.com/articles/whatisavegetarian.html.

Chapter 8: Sports Nutrition

America Dietetic Association. 2009. "Position of the American Dietetic Association: Nutrition and Athletic Performance." *Journal of the American Dietetic Association* 109(3): 509–527.

American Dietetic Association. www.eatright.org.

Clark, Nancy. 2008. *Nancy Clark's Sports Nutrition Guidebook*, 4th ed. Champaign, IL: Human Kinetics.

Coleman, E., and Steen, S. N. 2004. *Ultimate Sports Nutrition*, 2nd ed. Boulder: Bull Publishing Company.

Chapter 9: Funky Foods

About.com. "Most Popular Herbs and Supplements in the United States." http://altmedicine.about.com/library/weekly/aa022501a.htm.

American Dietetic Association. 2009. "Position of the American Dietetic Association: Functional Foods." *Journal of the American Dietetic Association* 109(4): 735–746.

Benefits of Resveratrol. "10 Super Foods & 10 Reasons to Eat These Super Foods." www.benefits-of-resveratrol.com/10-super-foods.html.

Botanical.com: A Modern Herbal. www.botanical.com.

Herbal Encyclopedia. "Safety with Herbs." www.naturalark.com/safety.html.

National Center for Complementary and Alternative Medicine. "Herbs at a Glance." http://nccam.nih.gov/health/herbsataglance.htm.

North American Institute of Medical Herbalism. http://medherb.com.

University of Texas–El Paso. "Herbal Safety." www.herbalsafety.utep.edu.

Zelman, K. 2008. "10 Everyday Super Foods." www.webmd.com/diet/guide/10-everyday-super-foods.

Chapter 10: Fast Facts on Fast Food

Burger King. "Menu and Nutrition." www.bk.com/en/us/menu-nutrition/index.html.

Chick-Fil-A. "Nutrition and Health." www.chick-fil-a.com/#nutrition.

Kentucky Fried Chicken. "Nutrition." www.kfc.com/nutrition/.

McDonalds. "Nutrition." www.mcdonalds.com/us/en/food/food_quality/nutrition_choices.html.

Starbucks. "Nutrition." www.starbucks.com/menu/nutrition.

Subway. "Nutritional Information." www.subway.com/applications/NutritionInfo/index.aspx.

Taco Bell. Nutrition Info. www.tacobell.com/nutrition.

Wendy's. Nutrition Facts. www.wendys.com/food/NutritionLanding.jsp.

Chapter 11: Meal Planning

2010 Dietary Guidelines Advisory Committee. "Meeting 6." 2010. www.cnpp.usda.gov/Publications/DietaryGuidelines/2010/Meeting6/DGAC Mtg6-Minutes-final.pdf.

Food and Nutrition Service. "National School Lunch Program." www.fns.usda.gov/cnd/lunch/.

Food and Safety Inspection Service. "Food Safety Education." www.fsis.usda.gov/Food_Safety_Education/index.asp.

Chapter 12: Cook It

Agricultural Marketing Service. "Understanding Organic Labeling." www.ams.usda.gov/AMSv1.0/ams.fetchTemplateData.do?template=Templat

eA&navID=NationalOrganicProgram&leftNav=NationalOrganic
Program&page=NOPUnderstandingOrganicLabeling&description
=Understanding%20Organic%20Labeling&acct=nopgeninfo

Clemson University Cooperative Extension. 2006. "Nutrition Claims on Food
Labels."
www.clemson.edu/extension/hgic/food/nutrition/nutrition/dietary_guide/hgi
c4061.html.

Food and Safety Inspection Service. "Food Safety Education."
www.fsis.usda.gov/Food_Safety_Education/index.asp.

Food Safety and Inspection Service. 2007. "Fact Sheet: Food Labeling: Food
Product Dating."
www.fsis.usda.gov/factsheets/food_product_dating/index.asp.

MindBodyGreen. 2010. "New 2010 List of 12 Fruits & Veggies with Highest
Amount of Pesticides: The 'Dirty Dozen'." www.mindbodygreen.com/
0-703/New-2010-List-of-12-Fruits-Veggies-with-Highest-Amount-of-Pesti-
cides-The-Dirty-Dozen.html.

MindBodyGreen. 2010. "New 2010 List of 15 Fruits & Veggies with Lowest
Amount of Pesticides: The 'Clean 15'." www.mindbodygreen.com/0-
704/New-2010-List-of-15-Fruits-Veggies-with-Lowest-Amount-of-Pesti-
cides-The-Clean-15.html.

U.S. Food and Drug Administration. 2003. "Claims That Can Be Made for Conventional Foods and Dietary Supplements."
www.fda.gov/Food/LabelingNutrition/LabelClaims/ucm111447.htm.

U.S. Food and Drug Administration. 2004. "How to Understand and Use the
Nutrition Facts Label."
www.fda.gov/food/labelingnutrition/consumerinformation/
ucm078889.htm.

U.S. Food and Drug Administration. 2009. "Background Information on Point
of Purchase Labeling."
www.fda.gov/Food/LabelingNutrition/LabelClaims/ucm187320.htm.

U.S. Food and Drug Administration. 2009. "New Front-of-Package Labeling Ini-
tiative." www.fda.gov/food/labelingnutrition/ucm202726.htm.

U.S. Food and Drug Administration. 2009. "Food Labeling Guide: Health
Claims." www.fda.gov/Food/GuidanceComplianceRegulatory
Information/GuidanceDocuments/FoodLabelingNutrition/FoodLabelingGui
de/ucm064919.htm.

U.S. Food and Drug Administration. 2010. "Labeling and Nutrition."
www.fda.gov/food/labelingnutrition/default.htm.

Index

Page numbers followed by a *t* indicate a table; numbers followed by a *f* indicate a figure.

A

Aerobic exercise, 48–49
Á la carte, 156
Alternative medicine, and herbal
    remedies, 114
Amino acids, 17–18, 87
    supplements, 109
Anemia, 41
Angel-devil smoothie, 184
Anorexia nervosa, 71
    behavior of people with, 76
    characteristics of people with, 76
    eating behaviors of, 72–73
    medical problems associated
        with, 78*t*
Antioxidants, 32, 45, 130
Appetite suppressants, 65*t*
Apple
    and oatmeal cookies, 242–243
    and peanut butter wedges, 233
    sauce, 227–228
    walnut crisp, 238–239
Artificial sweeteners, 16–17
Ascorbic acid. *See* Vitamin C
Aspartame, 16, 17
Athletes
    and dehydration, 101
    and eating disorders, 75

Athletes (cont'd)
    endurance, 111
    and fat intake, 100–101
    and protein intake, 99–100
    and snacking, 149
    and sport drinks, 103
    water intake requirements for,
        102
    and weight maintenance, 67, 69*t*

B

Banana
    bran muffins, 180–181
    shake, 185
Barley and mushroom risotto,
    187–188
Basal metabolic rate, 96, 111
Beans
    chowder, 191–192
    intake recommendations, 7*t*, 10
    pasta and, 210–211
    salad, 193
Beta-carotene, 45. *See also*
    Vitamin A
Beverage recipes
    Angel-devil smoothie, 184
    banana shake, 185
    fruit concoction, 186
Beverages
    comparison, 137*t*
    nutrition facts of some, 134–135
Binge eating disorder(BED), 72, 81